Special-Needs
Kids Go
Pharm-Free

Also by Judy Converse

SPECIAL-NEEDS KIDS EAT RIGHT:
STRATEGIES TO HELP KIDS ON THE AUTISM SPECTRUM FOCUS,
LEARN, AND THRIVE

Special-Needs Kids Go Pharm-Free

Nutrition-Focused Tools to Help Minimize Meds
and Maximize Health and Well-Being

Judy Converse, MPH, RD, LD

A PERIGEE BOOK

A PERIGEE BOOK
Published by the Penguin Group
Penguin Group (USA) Inc.
375 Hudson Street, New York, New York 10014, USA
Penguin Group (Canada), 90 Eglinton Avenue East, Suite 700, Toronto, Ontario M4P 2Y3, Canada
(a division of Pearson Penguin Canada Inc.)
Penguin Books Ltd., 80 Strand, London WC2R 0RL, England
Penguin Group Ireland, 25 St. Stephen's Green, Dublin 2, Ireland (a division of Penguin Books Ltd.)
Penguin Group (Australia), 250 Camberwell Road, Camberwell, Victoria 3124, Australia
(a division of Pearson Australia Group Pty. Ltd.)
Penguin Books India Pvt. Ltd., 11 Community Centre, Panchsheel Park, New Delhi—110 017, India
Penguin Group (NZ), 67 Apollo Drive, Rosedale, North Shore 0632, New Zealand
(a division of Pearson New Zealand Ltd.)
Penguin Books (South Africa) (Pty.) Ltd., 24 Sturdee Avenue, Rosebank, Johannesburg 2196,
South Africa
Penguin Books Ltd., Registered Offices: 80 Strand, London WC2R 0RL, England

While the author has made every effort to provide accurate telephone numbers and Internet addresses at the time of publication, neither the publisher nor the author assumes any responsibility for errors or for changes that occur after publication. Further, the publisher does not have any control over and does not assume any responsibility for author or third-party websites or their content.

Copyright © 2010 by Judy Converse, MPH, RD, LD
Text design by Tiffany Estreicher

First edition: December 2010

Library of Congress Cataloging-in-Publication Data

Converse, Judy.
    Special-needs kids go pharm-free : nutrition-focused tools to help minimize meds and maximize health and well-being / Judy Converse.— 1st ed.
        p.   cm.
    Includes index.
    ISBN 978-0-399-53622-9
    1. Diet therapy for children.   I. Title.
    RJ53.D53C66 2010
    618.92—dc22   2010035138

PRINTED IN THE UNITED STATES OF AMERICA

10   9   8   7   6   5   4   3   2   1

Neither the publisher nor the author is engaged in rendering professional advice or services to the individual reader. The ideas, procedures, and suggestions contained in this book are not intended as a substitute for consulting with your physician. All matters regarding your health require medical supervision. Neither the author nor the publisher shall be liable or responsible for any loss or damage allegedly arising from any information or suggestion in this book.

Most Perigee books are available at special quantity discounts for bulk purchases for sales promotions, premiums, fund-raising, or educational use. Special books, or book excerpts, can also be created to fit specific needs. For details, write: Special Markets, Penguin Group (USA) Inc., 375 Hudson Street, New York, New York 10014.

Contents

Nutrition Tools Help Many Special Situations for Kids

There are pages of helpful tips here that are now needed by more children than ever before. By 2005, nearly 13 percent of all U.S. children (some 9.3 million kids) were classifiable as having a special health care need, and this percentage has risen since then. Between 1980 and 2000, a 57 percent increase occurred in the rate of children with disabilities served by government programs. According to census data from 2000, one in twelve U.S. children (over 5 million kids) has a physical or mental disability. More current data from the Individuals with Disabilities Education Act (IDEA) estimates that a quarter of our children have a special need of some type, and show that the population of children served by IDEA programs has grown at more than twice the rate of the general education population, since the inception of IDEA in the 1970s. These are kids who need more than the usual medical care, who take a prescription medication on a daily basis, who have some diagnosed limitation to their functional abilities, or who re-quire ongoing physical, behavioral, occupational, or other therapy. Also included in that count are kids with chronic conditions such as asthma, diabetes, Crohn's disease, autism spectrum disorders, growth impairments, Down's syndrome, seizure disorders, ADHD, ADD, and food allergies.

These are kids who are at higher risk for nutrition problems, ac-cording to emerging research. As a dietitian in private practice, I have seen how profoundly a nutrition issue can impede a child, es-pecially children with special needs. Some data show that about 60 percent of all kids with special needs have nutrition problems. My guess is that this percentage may be even higher. In more than ten years in practice, I have rarely encountered a child who didn't have one. Worldwide, moderate to mild malnutrition—that is, the type I often see in practice here in the United States—causes significant increases in morbidity and mortality among children. Children with some type of special need comprise most of my practice, and it is common for them to come in with serious nutrition-related prob-lems that their pediatricians have missed.

What is "serious"? This can mean a variety of things. For example, a child has stopped growing as expected or stopped growing entirely; can't sleep, function, or focus; has frequent in-fections, in some cases necessitating long-term antibiotic use; has frequent bowel accidents at school and must stay home or has never had a normal bowel movement; is often sick and unable to stay well without antibiotics; or has behavior outbursts so disrup-tive that expulsion from school looms near and parents are at their wit's end; has persistent seizures, even with medication; has an ordinary flu that progresses to pneumonia and a hospital stay; has asthma events or food allergy reactions that whisk the child to the emergency room every month; has fluctuating blood sugar, close to a diabetes diagnosis; has suicidal thoughts; and so on. All these symptoms may have nutrition components that can create serious consequences if overlooked, undiagnosed, or untreated. Like any other piece to a puzzle, nutrition is rarely the whole story. Special-needs kids often need a team approach, including therapies for learning, physical issues, and emotional health. Good nutrition, too, should be part of your child's team, and not impeding the progress he or she deserves.

Parents come to me looking for options beyond pharmaceuticals to help their kids feel, function, and grow better. They do this for varied reasons. Often, a pharmaceutical path has failed (for example, their child cannot be weaned off laxatives or proton pump inhibitors, without worsening reflux and constipation; or she's taking a stimulant but is still struggling with attention and focus). Other parents simply want to learn more about natural approaches before using drugs. As a licensed nutrition professional, I use nutrition-focused tools, and I choose these based on a thoughtful, individualized assessment of each child. Any parent can access this care by requesting a referral from their pediatrician to a licensed nutrition professional, or by working with a licensed naturopathic doctor; some insurances may cover the care. Nutrition-focused tools can work very well—examples from my practice include weaning a clinically depressed teen entirely off an antidepressant medication that was doing little good and replacing it with a successful natural protocol; reducing or eliminating the need for daily steroids and anti-inflammatories in a child with asthma; or reversing failure to thrive in a toddler already using growth hormone injections. While I have often seen nutrition-focused tools supersede the need for pharmaceuticals entirely, I also work with children who need and successfully use pharmaceuticals, and I engage a child's MD care team in this process either way. The two modalities can work nicely together, as long as you have a care team willing to communicate with each other. Whichever route you take with your child, this book offers supports and information to help you along the way.

If a child could benefit more from a nutrition-focused tool than a pharmaceutical one, your pediatrician may not know about it. In the United States, medical doctors aren't required to take thorough training in nutrition or complementary and alternative therapies, as they are in some other countries. Though there is ongoing review of nutrition-focused strategies in academic litera-ture, many doctors don't have time to read about it all. Even if they did, they may not be getting the straight scoop. Later in this book you will read about a study that found some venerable med-ical journals to be biased against nonpharmaceutical treatments.

Another hurdle that physicians encounter in providing families with information about nutrition strategies is their contracts with the health insurers who pay them for your child's visits. These contracts dictate how much the doctor is paid for the visit, based on the diagnosis and procedure codes the doctor assigns to it. They also will state preferred prescribing practices; some medications will be preferentially covered over others. Pharmaceutical compa-nies that offer incentives to doctors for prescribing certain medi-cines have been scrutinized (and criticized) far and wide, from places such as the nation's capital in congressional hearings, to a variety of journals, books, and websites. Conflicts of interest aside, if your pediatrician is not up to speed on nutrition screening, as-sessment, or diagnosis coding, getting the right care for a nutrition problem can be a challenge. This is "managed care" in the United

States today. Health insurers and pharmaceutical companies don't sell healthy eating habits, nutrition referrals, supplements, nutraceuticals, or herbal remedies. That's because these are mostly unpatentable (and thus, a lot less profitable than a drug); there are no contracts with insurers to price and sell these; and it takes many more minutes in a doctor's visit to discuss and give instructions on nutrition than it takes to use a prescription pad.

Because of these realities in medicine today, a pediatrician must make a particular effort to practice beyond the prescription pad. Raising healthy kids also requires some extra effort from parents who are interested in safe tools that don't require a prescription. Changes to help our kids be healthier can't come soon enough: For the first time in history, U.S. children are expected to have a shorter life span than their parents. More than any generation before them in America, kids today already have chronic disability and disease. At younger ages and with an alarming frequency never seen before, *children* have cancer, leukemia, diabetes, asthma, life-threatening allergies, inflammatory bowel disease, Crohn's disease—not to mention devastating developmental delays such as autism, global and pervasive developmental delays, learning disabilities, and behavior and mood problems bad enough to keep them out of school. Despite more options for children than ever before from the pharmaceutical industry, more doctors' visits annually than in years past, and more prescription drug use than ever among children, our children are doing more poorly, according to data from private and government sources.

Pharmaceuticals rarely fix nutrition problems. In my experience, just as the data has shown, most special-needs kids have nutrition problems, which can improve with nutrition-focused tools. Nutrition problems make children sick more often, cause a harsher course of illness when they do get sick, trigger learning and behavior issues, and increase risk for chronic diseases. Nutrition deficits in kids are linked in thousands of research articles to behavior, sleep, learning, growth, weight gain, development, brain function, mood, and more. You can safely leverage nutrition-focused tools to help your child reach his potential for health, growth, and functioning. This means using diet, foods, and/or supplements instead of, before, or alongside pharmaceutical strategies. Supplements can include essential nutrients, probiotics, herbs, or nonessential nutrients that show efficacy for certain problems (such as adding coenzyme Q10, a nonessential nutritive supplement, to what are called "mito cocktails" for children with mitochondrial disorder). The options are almost unlimited, and waiting to be tapped.

Americans spent nearly $300 *billion* on medications in 2008, and this was considered a down year by the pharmaceutical industry, owing to the slowed economy. Clearly, the financial motivation to access the pediatric population is compelling for this industry, which expects annual growth. In 2008, antipsychotic medications took the lead for overall prescription sales. For children, stimulant drugs (such as Ritalin) and antidepressants by far outpace prescriptions for other drugs. Is this safe, necessary, or effective? These are decisions to make carefully with your pediatric MD providers. Children should be thoughtfully assessed and diagnosed by a pediatric specialist before a prescription is given. Many drugs are used "off label" in children—that is, they are used in age groups and for conditions for which they have not been approved by the FDA. If you aren't certain that your pediatrician has all the information you need, ask for a referral to a specialist who is experienced in prescribing for children.

Meanwhile, use this book to discern which nutrition tools to try when. These can be safe, effective, and tend to have beneficial rather than negative side effects—for example, one clinical trial found that children with autism who are given melatonin not only slept better, but experienced fewer and less intense obsessive-compulsive behaviors during the day. Explore these unsung options, and engage your pediatric providers in the conversation. Our children are challenged like never before, and deserve the best we can give to optimize their health and functioning. For more help, information, resources, and support, visit my website at NutritionCare.net.

Chapter One

Special-Needs Babies

NOT WHAT YOU EXPECTED

Why include a chapter in this book on babies, when the last thing you want to think about at the start of your child's life is whether he will be delayed or impaired in some way, or have a serious health challenge? Here's why: Some babies enter the world with quite a bang. They show up early and suddenly, and need lots of help to stay with us. Others come when expected, healthy and well, only to insidiously slip into a quagmire of problems with feeding, eliminating, growing, sleeping, and exploring as babies need to do. At this early point in your child's life, the truth in either case is that nutrition has profound and lasting impacts. You can leverage it at this young moment to set him up for years of better health, learning, growth, and development. After years of taking life histories on special-needs children, I can tell you that this *does* matter. Your child may avoid or be less affected by conditions such as asthma, diabetes, severe allergies, chronic illness, or learning and developmental problems by using nutrition-focused strategies early on.

When my husband and I started our family, I was already a nutritionist, so I knew this. Odd as it sounds, it took me a while to realize that other parents did *not* know this. I assumed they would have an inkling about it, because I assumed that pediatricians had to know and apply tenets of child nutrition in practice. Mostly, they don't. It stunned me that parents could not get more than basic information from their pediatricians about nutrition. As it turned out in my case, I needed more than that. This is what redirected me into doing the work I have done now for more than a decade.

Here's a bit of advice I was given during pregnancy by a well-meaning older parent: "Babies are so easy. You don't need to buy a bunch of stuff or even a crib. You could just put them in a drawer with some cotton batting. They are easy and don't need anything, just cuddles and feeding." Another friend (no kids) told me that having a dog was crucial to proper parenting and raising normal kids. At eight months pregnant and feeling like heavy furniture, the last thing I wanted was to train a new puppy. Why do people with the least experience give the most advice?

What parents of typically developing, healthy, and able children may not realize is that a good measure of the success they enjoy in child rearing is due to luck. When infants are lucky enough to have ordinary, normal feeding skills, food tolerance, digestion, growth, development, sleep patterns, and eliminations, they usually *are* pretty easy to care for. This does not require perfection parenting. It is easy to take care of a baby when he has a healthy, stable constitution; no birth defects; no conditions or circumstances interfering with normal structure and function of that pristine little body. Babies generally do begin sleeping in longer stretches, relatively soon, when they are well. They grow fast, chub up, look around, smile, recover fast from bumps or frights, and explore. They take to solid foods with curiosity, steady growth, and normal stools. They don't spend most of their time breathlessly screaming or filling their clothes with sour vomit or their diapers with mucousy, liquid stools.* They don't stare vacantly for hours when they are awake; they do contentedly explore with their newly noted fingers, toes, or mouths rather than avoid the world. No one signs on for seizure disorders, growth failure, micropremie status, developmental delays, meningitis, or cystic fibrosis in a baby. These and even lesser problems naturally make parents anxious, which can in turn upset their baby even more. When arduous challenges like these come your way, gathering information from sources that bolster and empower you is a top priority.

Over the course of my years in practice, many parents tell me that they have had to reach past the usual baby books, the pediatrician, or even their regional children's hospital for answers. Others have told me how they have been made to feel responsible for their baby's health problems, when no strategies to fix the problem were offered. Help may be somewhere else entirely for families of special-needs kids. You need family, respite, friends, and health care providers who can support you as a parent, and guide your family to grow up strong. If your baby is facing challenges beyond the typical, tips in this chapter tell you how to use

---

* It is not normal or benign for an infant to experience a persisting pattern of explosive wet stool; copious stool that soils the baby's legs, back, and neck; or dry, hard stools that are painful to pass. These signal malabsorption or possibly a stomach bug.

nutritional supports, and how to talk to your doctors about it—whether your little one is at home or in the NICU. Here's some advice to start, better than telling you to get a puppy and some cotton batting:

- There are no dumb questions, so don't ever hesitate to ask your providers for more information, referrals, or possible alternate strategies if your baby isn't progressing as expected. Your doctor works for *you*. If your child isn't thriving or evolving under his or her care, if your doctor is a poor listener, or if someone on your care team leaves you feeling humiliated, frightened, or hopeless, it's time to change doctors.

- Moms. Know. Best. I have very rarely seen this *not* to be the case. A parent's intuition is a powerful thing, and while there may or may not be research to back this up, it seems to grow with the pregnancy and the job—and somehow sticks around just about forever. Listen to it and permit it to guide you to the solutions, professional supports, and tools that just might be best for your baby.

- Nutrition and food are the cornerstone of health for infants, period. Making sure your baby eats and absorbs her diet adequately and comfortably ensures the best platform for growth, development, and robust immune function.

No matter what circumstances your baby has, normal and adequate nutrient assimilation is the single most important driver of his health outcome, for years to come. It is what permits your baby's brain, body, and immune system to exist, grow, and function. This often gets overlooked in modern pediatrics, where the focus is on immunization schedules at each "well baby" visit. But humans can't have immune systems at all without the nutrients to build them, and babies can fail quickly with even slight nutrition deficits. Babies are exquisitely sensitive to nutrition deficits, to inflammation from feedings, or to infections and illness. Make sure their immune and digestive functions are as robust as possible with these steps.

Start with Food—and Bacteria?

What your baby eats and how she absorbs it is her foundation for everything. But before we go there, equal time should be given to another part of the puzzle on how babies grow, function, develop, and acquire normal immune function. New research is emerging about an interesting choreography between humans and the bacteria we encounter at birth. It turns out that babies whose intestines are populated early with certain microflora—that is, bacteria—have better long-term health outcomes, less asthma, and fewer allergies than babies whose intestines never establish this healthy profile of bacterial residents. These benefits last throughout childhood, and even throughout life. Circumstances that disturb this for babies are C-section delivery, early and frequent use of antibiotics (for Mom at delivery, while nursing, or for baby), procedures necessitating surgeries that include antibiotics, or premie status.

Since the 1980s, infants and children have been dosed with antibiotics and vaccines much more frequently than they were before. Both of these tools—which together comprise much of pediatric care today—can interfere with normal bowel microflora. In the same time frame, asthma, diabetes, obesity, neurodevelopmental disorders, and life-threatening food allergies have skyrocketed in children. Research suggests that this early interplay between helpful microbes and the human gut plays a crucial role in teaching our immune systems how to function smoothly. To assess this, I often request stool cultures on infants, toddlers, and children in my practice, and use a lab that cultures both beneficial and detrimental strains. My clinical experience concurs with the emerging research: Babies and kids are healthier, grow better, have fewer inflammatory conditions such as food allergies and asthma, and eat a healthier, more varied diet when they establish healthy bowel flora in the first two years of life. When they encounter an early circumstance such as C-section, premie birth, time in the NICU with antibiotics, frequent infections with more antibiotics—these are the kids who have more allergies, inflammation, asthma, bowel problems, and challenging growth and eating patterns as they grow up. These are the kids in my caseload who also tend to have more learning, developmental, and behavior problems.

It's clear that setting up healthy intestinal function from birth is linked to long-term health outcomes. Some research has supported this in findings that bacteria ingested during early infancy are more likely to permanently colonize the intestine than those ingested later on in childhood, a scenario I witness often in practice. It looks like this: Many school-age children I encounter can't seem to keep normal, healthy intestinal flora (and appetite, behavior, or bowel function) without maintenance regimens of drugs such as Flagyl, Bactram, or Diflucan. These are strong drugs that kill fungal species and bacteria normally controlled by our own immune function and bowel microflora. Even when given these drugs *and* high-potency probiotics, these kids' stool cultures sometimes still lack beneficial strains. When they go off these drugs and probiotics, these kids worsen dramatically for bowel function and behavior. Invariably, these are children whose early months and years included circumstances that egregiously disturbed colonization of the gut with normal microflora. Children who have more minor interruptions in early colonization of good microflora seem to be able to rebound later on, if dosed correctly with probiotics and other nutrition measures.

Special circumstances for babies often necessitate tools such as antibiotics, or giving formula or breast milk to babies born before term, when their feeding and digestive functions are fragile. Probiotics can be extremely helpful in these circumstances. The colonization process for a baby's gut begins right at birth, when the sterile, germ-free womb is left behind. This process is also influenced by Mom's own microflora, and by type of feeding: Formula-fed infants have lower counts of beneficial bacteria than breast-fed infants. Heavier colonization of beneficial strains such as bifidobacteria species have also been associated with better overall health in babies.

It's easy to add beneficial microflora to your baby's intake. These are sold as probiotic supplements, that is, powdered blends of "colony forming units" (CFUs). These are live, viable bacteria that have an identifiable, positive impact on health. Probiotics are a common intervention for babies and children outside the United States, where they are often prescribed over other measures for diarrhea, colic, and irritable or inflammatory bowel diseases. Researchers have studied several individual strains that are beneficial to humans. There are countless other strains to learn about, and this will likely become a niche in medicine unto itself in the near future. Fermented foods contain probiotics naturally, and these may be added after about age eight to ten months, depending on your baby's circumstances.

When and how should you consider probiotics for a baby? What products are best? Here are situations that warrant this measure:

Premature birth. If your premie is having trouble getting settled on a good feeding, sleeping, and growth pattern, probiotics could be a piece of the puzzle. Microflora such as bifidobacteria, *Streptococcus thermophilus*, and some lactobacillus species can help your baby digest food, crowd out pathogens, and signal the immune system away from unnecessary inflammatory responses.

C-section birth. Babies born this way miss the benefit of traveling down the birth canal, where exposure to Mom's vaginal microflora starts them off on the right foot for imprinting the intestine with good bacteria. (Mom will want to avoid vaginal yeast infections and remain healthy during pregnancy.) They may also have had an exposure to antibiotics, when Mom receives them via IV with surgery. Antibiotics given to Mom postsurgery to prevent wound infection will also be in her milk, and her baby will receive them if she breast-feeds. Though the American Academy of Pediatrics' standard is to defer vaccination when a child is sick with a fever, and thus likely to be prescribed an antibiotic, babies are routinely vaccinated at birth, even though they may be exposed to antibiotics at the same time. The long-term effects of this on the development of the immune system are unstudied. You can help your baby's immune function and digestion by using gentle probiotics.

Necrotizing enterocolitis. One of the problems often encountered by low-birth-weight or premature babies is necrotizing enterocolitis (NEC). This means that the wall of the baby's bowel becomes inflamed to such an extent that it is damaged, and this tender new gut tissue can die. NEC is serious, with a significant mortality rate. The lower the baby's weight, the higher the risk for a poor outcome with NEC. Many causes for NEC have been considered, and it appears that abnormal intestinal microflora is among them. If your baby has NEC, your care team should include a probiotic supplement in the care plan. If possible, breast milk should be considered over formula, since this will help populate your baby's gut with the most beneficial species of bacteria. Breast-fed babies have NEC less often than formula-fed babies; not only do they have more beneficial microbes growing in their intestines when breast-fed, but they have less of a diarrhea-causing bacteria caused clostridia. Human milk has a sugar in it called oligofructose, and this helps the right bacteria grow in the intestine. Formula without this sugar causes more clostridia to grow. If you can't breast-feed and your care team can't provide formula with ingredients to help good bacteria grow, consider using breast milk from a milk bank. Contact the National Milk Bank or ask your hospital care team about this option.

Antibiotics in infancy. Though we use antibiotics often in infants, and they are lifesaving when necessary, using them may come with a price. The immune function of mucosa that line the throat and GI tract is undeveloped in babies, making those mucosal surfaces more permeable. This makes babies more susceptible to infections because pathogens have an easier time penetrating those tissues than they do in adults and older children. Inflammation at those mucosal tissues is tougher on an infant, too; it can cause structural damage and more permeability. Probiotics appear to reduce inflammation, and thus help mucosa in the gut and throat stay healthy. When the beneficial bacteria they deliver get established, they can crowd out infectious pathogens. They literally tighten up the intestinal wall, and make it less permeable. Some beneficial bacteria excrete acids that can kill infectious microbes, too. So if your baby has needed antibiotics, it's helpful to follow with a course of probiotics. Continue them for at least twice as long as the time your baby was on an antibiotic. Typically, I suggest babies in my practice use probiotics for at least three months after even brief courses of antibiotic treatments, to restore normal bowel flora.

Eczema. Babies with eczema or heavy cradle cap may be struggling to digest their feedings. If this is the case, it is likely a protein intolerance. Many providers and parents alike confuse this with lactose intolerance, and waste time using lactose-free formulas. Lactose is the sugar in milk, not the protein, and while it may cause some digestive upset or gas, this typically occurs in older children or adults, not babies. Babies who truly can't digest lactose or its smaller sugar components quickly falter and fail to thrive. If this is the case, a specialized formula without milk or lactose is required (your pediatrician may screen for galactosemia, an inherited disorder in which no milk- or lactose-containing products are tolerated). Premature babies sometimes do not have enough enzymes to digest lactose; in these cases, milk-free formulas are useful. In any case, lactose intolerance does not have eczema—an inflammatory response—among its symptoms. Diarrhea, gas, stomach pain, and bloating are typical with lactose intolerance. These may occur with milk protein intolerance as well, but when eczema enters the picture, this is confirming of an inflammatory response that lactose doesn't trigger, but proteins do.

Your baby will need a formula change if she has persisting eczema. If a baby is on cow's milk formula, I often recommend a "semi-elemental" one such as Nutramigen or Alimentum, or a partly digested one such as Carnation Good Start. Some babies may fare well on soy formula, and it may be worth a shot before other formulas are tried. But in my experience, soy formula is often just as troublesome as cow's milk formula for babies. If you've switched to soy formula and your baby seems better at first only to slip into worsening symptoms after a week or two, then your baby's immune system is likely reacting to soy protein now as well. I recommend trying the semi-elemental formulas next. If these fail, I usually suggest moving to an elemental infant formula such as Neocate.

If you are breast-feeding and your baby struggles with eczema, colic, and frequent diarrhea, consider a trial of semi-elemental or elemental formulas to see if symptoms improve. If they do, this is confirming that your breast milk is not well tolerated by your baby. As difficult as weaning before you'd hoped can be, it's important to know that reducing inflammation in your baby's gut will permit better nutrient absorption, better growth, and less frequent illness. In this scenario, a probiotic can help make up for the loss of some of the beneficial effects of your breast milk.

Some moms commit to nursing through these tough signs and symptoms by restricting their own food intakes to exclude suspected trigger foods for the baby. As a nutritionist, I felt especially firm about giving my baby breast milk. While his symptoms improved on a trial of semi-elemental formula, I still wanted him to have all the benefits of breast milk. I needed to follow a very restricted diet to keep his symptoms to a dull roar. It was exhausting, and I depleted myself doing this. If you are breast-feeding, you need good-quality nutrition to make enough milk while keeping your own bones, hair, skin, gums, sleep cycle, mood, and energy levels healthy. Removing more than five or six foods from your diet to accommodate your nursing baby can start to become too injurious to *you* to really be sustainable. The quality of your breast milk won't vary much—your body will produce the best milk it can at any cost. But the amount you can produce may drop if you are too depleted, and the cost to your own physical well-being can become too high. If you are feeling exhausted and depleted, sleeping poorly, losing hair quickly, feeling irritable or depressed most of the time, or notice changes in your skin or nails, then you are depleting yourself too much. See the resources section of this book for tips on taking care of yourself as a new mom, and making sure your own nutrition stays strong.

Babies who have eczema appear to have a "disturbed" intestinal barrier, in the words of Tanmeet Sethi, MD, who reviewed probiotics in an article called "Probiotics in Pediatric Care" (published in *Explore* in 2009). The right microflora work to restore normal health and function of that barrier. The strains of beneficial bacteria that have shown promise for relieving eczema symptoms are *Lactobacillus rhamnosus* and *Lactobacillus reuteri*. These were tested in a double-blind, placebo-controlled, randomized study (published in the *Lancet* in 2001), and other studies since have delivered good news on probiotics and eczema. A product such as Klaire Labs Therbiotic Infant Formula contains these strains, as well as bifidobacteria species that normally populate a baby's gut.

Tube feedings. If your baby is receiving a formula through a feeding tube, talk with your care team about putting a probiotic in the feeding. Formula shifts intestinal microflora away from a more beneficial profile compared to breast milk, and circumstances necessitating the tube probably injured your baby's microflora establishment also—so this is a perfect storm of circumstances that can deter normal microflora colonies from growing, and an important opportunity to restore them. While probiotics have a pristine safety record, at least two events describing probiotic bacteremia and sepsis have been published (an astronomically better safety record than medicines or vaccines); these occurred in high-risk infants who were on feeding tubes. Check with your care team before adding a probiotic to the feeding tube, and have your doctor help you choose carefully which ones to use. Bifidobacteria species, and lactobacillus strains such as *rhamnosus* and *reuteri*, seem well tolerated in babies, but any live bacteria given to excess has the potential to be injurious. Have your care team check the latest research on what works best, in terms of chosen strains and potency of probiotic. Don't buy over-the-counter products for adults and put them in your baby's feeding tube. Besides possibly having the wrong strains for your baby's needs, they may have other ingredients your baby doesn't need, such as fillers, starches, or additional nutrients.

Cystic fibrosis. I don't have many children with cystic fibrosis in my caseload, since these kids routinely access nutrition care through their major medical centers (unlike kids with autism, developmental delays, asthma, or severe food allergies, who may get spotty to no nutrition assessment, monitoring, or care). But there are still a few tricks to mention for CF kids. Cystic fibrosis is an inflammatory condition affecting some 30,000 persons in the United States. Its hallmark is inflammation and excessive mucus production in lung, intestinal, and reproductive tissue. Probiotics have been shown to reduce intestinal inflammation in cystic fibrosis. Babies with cystic fibrosis should also be given the least inflammatory food or formula. This may mean using a specialized baby formula that is "elemental" if breast milk is not well tolerated. Virtually all the nutrients in an elemental formula are ready to absorb, and require no or minimal digestion. The protein source in an elemental formula is ready to absorb, too. Instead of using protein from soy or casein, elemental formulas use individual amino acids as a protein source. Amino acids are what proteins are made of; when a protein is digested in our intestines, it ends up as individual free amino acids, which are then absorbed. Along with using probiotics, elemental protein sources like this can also reduce inflammation.

A final word of advice for CF babies who have excess mucus—especially when mucus is seen in vomit or stool or is backing up into a gastrectomy tube—is to consider enzymes that break mucus apart. One enzyme product specifically designed for this is called Mucostop. This and other enzyme products may help break apart the "biofilm" that builds in the gut, which may build up even more in CF babies, or kids with chronic GI problems. Biofilm is a matrix of mucus, fungus, viral material, or other disruptive microbial species that surrounds itself with a gelatinous goop in order to make itself impenetrable to just about anything. It makes normal digestion and absorption from the intestine pretty difficult and can exacerbate constipation. Breaking this up with tools such as Mucostop, ViraStop, Candidase (Enzymedica), Candex (Pure Essence), or strong-potency enzymes for protein digestion may help. Digestive enzymes for food may be useful as well, since CF can hinder our own production and secretion of these. Your doctor may prescribe a digestive enzyme. If this is poorly tolerated, review high-potency nonprescription enzyme products from reputable companies (such as Enzymedica, Houston Enzymes, or Kirkman Labs) with your provider. To assure appropriate use of their products, many makers of higher-end supplements make them available only through health care providers, so you may not see the products you need on store shelves. If your MD provider is unfamiliar with these tools, ask a licensed naturopathic doctor (ND) for input.

Colic. There's colic, and then there's *colic*. A little fussing now and then is one thing. But when babies lose most of every feeding with projectile vomiting or spoonfuls of spit-up, and slip down their growth charts because of it, stop struggling—it's time to take action. Colic usually also includes hard, bulging tummies that are full of painful gas, crying upon being placed in a supine position for sleep after a feeding, or only being able to sleep upright. You may also see copious stools that are yellow, wet, foul, and mucousy (these are markedly different from normal breast-fed stools, which may be more gold than brown and wet or soft, but not mucousy, explosive, runny, or foul smelling). This is not benign for your baby, and this is not a "cry it out" moment. Colic can keep a baby in distress and pain. Leaving your baby to cry himself to sleep while in pain is cruel. Stools as I've described here are not benign either—they signal malabsorption and inflammation, or possibly infection with destructive microflora.

If colic is not an issue, your baby will probably cry relatively briefly for a few nights, then learn to fall asleep alone with little fanfare. If it is an issue, no amount of abandonment will make the underlying problem go away. Change formulas; switch off breast milk if you must, or change your own diet while nursing; and add probiotics. You might even try some gentle digestive herbs that are safe for babies (described in Chapter 2). In fact, one of the least effective things you can do is medicate colic with tools such as Mylicon (simethicone) drops. These drops simply help gas bubbles stick to each other so that larger and larger bubbles form, and become easier to release out one end of your baby or the other— but simethicone drops don't address why your baby is making so much gas, or reduce its production. Research reviews have shown simethicone drops to be least effective in reducing colic in babies, compared to changing feeding sources or using herbs. See Chapter 2 for more information on using herbs for babies with colic.

Thrush. This is a fungal infection that babies can get in their mouths or diaper area; it may occur on Mom's nipples also, if you and your baby exchange thrush between breast and mouth. It looks like white velvety or fuzzy patches on tongue, gums, anus, or genitals; sometimes patches will appear in stools. Under the patches on mucus membranes, tissue may be red and may bleed easily. Thrush is caused by candida (fungal) overgrowth, and there are many strains of candida and other fungal species that can infect a human gut. A bit of these residing there isn't usually a problem; normally, they are kept in check by our own healthy microflora. But candida (aka "yeast") will flourish when our own immune defenses are weak, when antibiotics clear out beneficial microflora, or in conditions such as AIDS or diabetes.

Thrush is often treated with drugs such as Nystatin or Diflucan in babies. Probiotics are useful follow-ups to those medications when babies have thrush, to ensure that healthy microflora are taking residence in the GI tract. Even if no antifungal medication was prescribed, your baby may need one anyway, if there are troubling symptoms such as explosive or foul stools, diarrhea, or constipated stools. These signs indicate (in my experience) that intestinal candida overgrowth is persisting, even if thrush is no longer visible at the mouth or diaper area. High-potency probiotics (above 12 billion CFUs per day) can conquer thrush and intestinal candidiasis in some cases, eliminating the need for drug treatments. Older children may need as much as 50 billion CFUs of a probiotic blend daily to make headway on entrenched candida infections. Troubleshoot this with your provider team, and seek help from those experienced with using probiotics. Children vary for which strains and potencies they may need or tolerate best.

Diarrhea and constipation. Babies, like everybody else, need to move their bowels daily. Stool that sits in the intestine and colon for too long permits toxins to flow back into circulation, can feel painful or uncomfortable, and can diminish your baby's appetite. Stool that passes too fast will carry too much fluid out with it, and nutrients and energy won't be adequately absorbed. More than anyone else, babies are quite sensitive to these dilemmas. Occasional changes in this pattern are of no consequence; persisting patterns are. This is common sense as much as it is sensible nutrition science. Many things disrupt stooling for babies. Teething, stress, immunizations, antibiotics, badly tolerated foods, and infections or illnesses can all trigger changes in stooling pattern, but the changes should be *temporary*. Even if your baby is struggling with special circumstances, endeavor to restore as typical a digestive function as you can. On balance, your baby should comfortably pass one or two formed soft stools every day (perhaps up to four if breast-feeding), and it shouldn't smell terrible. Breast-fed infants have softer, mushier, wetter stools that look more seedy and light brown or gold, and these babies may pass stools more often. Younger babies may also have more frequent stools. But if any of the following signs persist for more than two or three weeks with no explanation, consider it a flag for distressed digestion and absorption, and make a plan to correct it:

- More than four stools per day

- Liquid, runny, or watery stools

- Mucus in stools

- Undigested food in stools

- Stools that are explosive or overflow onto your baby's back or neck

- Yellow, gold, tan, pale gray, black, or green stools (dark mustard–colored stools are normal for breast-fed infants)

- Blood in stools

- No stools passed for more than three days on a regular basis

- Hard, dry, pebble-like stool that appears painful or difficult to pass

- Plugs of hard stool followed by explosive loose stool

- Unusually foul-smelling stools

Probiotics are one of the corrections you will want to use to restore a healthy stool pattern, and they may be the only one you need. Generally, these guidelines for giving probiotics to babies can help; if you aren't sure, check with a provider who has experience using them:

- Place ⅛ teaspoon of bifidobacteria blend probiotic powder in your baby's feeding once a day. If this is tolerated and no improvements ensue, increase to ¼ teaspoon.

- Stop if you notice explosive diarrhea, hives, fever, or sudden rashes.

- Look for bifidobacteria strains such as *B. breve, B. infantis, B. longum,* and *B. bifidum* in the product, and a potency of at least 8 billion CFUs per dose.

- Safe lactobacillus strains that can be added for babies nearing their first birthday or for toddlers are *L. rhamnosus, L. casei, L. paracasei, L. gasseri, L. reuteri,* and *L. salvarius.*

- Don't use *L. acidophilus* for babies, premies, or infants with NEC. The form of lactic acid made by this species appears to be tolerated poorly in babies. In fact, one study showed that it actually increased allergy (noted as skin rashes) in babies.

- Probiotic powder can be blended with soft food, breast milk, or formula. You can also dust some on the nipple of the bottle or the breast.

- Infants should avoid probiotic strains and blends that are intended for adults.

- Don't give probiotics at the same time as an antibiotic. The antibiotic will kill the probiotic. Wait until the course of antibiotic is completed, then begin using a probiotic daily.

- If your baby must use antibiotics for longer than two weeks or indefinitely, you can add probiotics at the opposite end of the day. For example, if an antibiotic is given in the morning, give the probiotics in the afternoon or evening.

Reflux and how it relates to diarrhea, constipation, and colic. As I've mentioned, these are not benign for a baby. Persisting in the absence of obvious causes, they signal malabsorption, overgrowth of detrimental bowel microflora, inflammation, or all three. These three problems may exacerbate or trigger reflux in babies. Giving reflux medication may allow quick reprieve from symptoms, but using it longer than a few weeks may set a downward spiral in motion. Reflux medications can alter pH of the GI tract in favor of candida, other fungal species, or detrimental bacteria such as klebsiella or clostridia. These microbes produce toxins of their own, which further alter the gut's pH, and which can cross the blood-brain barrier to alter behavior. In turn, this impairs digestion and absorption more, because our own digestive enzymes and hormones are most effective in a narrow pH range.

I have encountered babies who have gotten "stuck" on reflux medication, needing increasingly higher doses that become less and less effective. One whom I encountered was given reflux medication daily for the first three years of his life. Though he had been off this medication for three years by the time I met him at age six, he was stunted with delayed bone age and poor bone mineralization, growth failure, developmental and learning problems, and was unable to eat enough to sustain normal growth since eating was so uncomfortable. He'd had chronic infections as an infant and toddler, needed antibiotics often, and became asthmatic as well. Another youngster who came in for nutrition care at age three was also stuck on it, had fallen into growth failure, and showed the same pattern of not being able to achieve a typical food intake to support growth and gain. Many other toddlers I have met show this pattern of growth failure owing to picky, weak appetites after using reflux medications for a long time (more than a month or two). Reflux medications are intended for short-term symptomatic treatment, not as a long-term strategy. You may have more success by trying the corrections described here first instead, so discuss them with your provider. Your baby will be healthier and will grow and feel better if digestion can evolve normally rather than with chronic down-regulation from the medication strategy.

When stool changes described above persist for weeks and months, nutrients and energy are not being absorbed as intended by your baby, and unintended toxins can be absorbed. Babies who are showing negative changes in their growth patterns amid these symptoms are sending an additional, especially clear signal that you need to intervene. Don't wait for your baby to slide into a failure-to-thrive (FTT) diagnosis, which means less than the 5th percentile in weight for age. Babies in growth failure need two to three times more calories per pound per day to recover a normal growth pattern, and this is even more challenging to accomplish when a baby has reflux or other GI issues. Intervene as soon as you notice a "dropping-off channel"—that is, if your baby's weight for age or length for age percentile drops more than fifteen points, it's time to intervene.

Besides incorporating a probiotic, you will probably need to change formula or feeding strategy if your baby's stools are as described above, or if there is hard colic, vomiting, reflux, or lots of spit-up. These two measures alone may stop your baby's reflux, and I have witnessed this many times. If these don't do the trick, obtain a stool culture for your baby that will screen for fungal species. Use a test for bacteria and yeast culture and sensitivities that can identify and quantify individual microbial strains. It should also identify what medications and herbs killed your child's fungal and bacterial cultures. This lets your MD provider prescribe a medication if necessary, with confidence that it can do the job. You can work with herbs suggested on the sensitivity panel, too. I have repeatedly seen antifungal therapy, via both herbal and prescription tools, eradicate reflux, constipation, and diarrhea in infants.

Changing formulas or feeding strategies. Don't persist with a formula or food that is making your baby miserable—and if you see signs mentioned in this chapter for odd stools, your baby is probably not feeling too well. And don't persist with breast milk either if your baby is not growing as expected or tolerating it well. Breast milk is without peer; it is what babies need, and in the vast majority of cases should have. Many texts, websites, and research articles eloquently deliver the scientific discourse on why this is true. But there are circumstances that can make even this perfect food hard for a baby to absorb. I probably never would say this if I had not gone through it myself as a parent; my training in public health nutrition under at least two graduate advisors who were militant breast-feeding advocates would never permit it. But contrary to my training with these smart women, my own son could not tolerate breast milk, and after six months of exhausting and depleting myself with restricted diets and watching him grow weakly, I threw in the towel.

Breast milk can contain cow's milk protein fragments when Mom's diet is rich in dairy foods, or fragments from any food protein that Mom eats. These may trigger inflammation or colicky symptoms in your baby. Stories abound of foods Mom eats changing a baby's symptoms. After eating a lot of pecans and walnuts on my heavily restricted diet while nursing, these became the only nuts to which my son acquired a hives reaction, even though he has never eaten them himself. If you are breast-feeding and your baby has colic, try removing casein and whey (milk protein) sources to see if this improves things. Don't replace cow's milk products with soy products. Infants who don't tolerate cow's milk protein frequently have the same trouble with soy. Soy also interferes with absorption of some minerals, especially iron. Fermented soy products such as miso and tempeh are easier to digest and absorb, and will interfere less with mineral absorption. See the resources section for more strategies on nourishing yourself while you are nourishing your baby.

If this just all gets to be too much, as was true in my own case as a new mom, then what? Certainly try semi-elemental and elemental formulas; your pediatrician will be informed about these. After trials with a number of commercial formulas failed in my own son's case, I actually created a formula recipe for him using powdered, pasteurized goat milk. This was in 1997, when the Internet had marginal functionality and content. So I cracked open my old textbooks, worked through science and medical libraries, contacted old friends from graduate school, and figured it out. It worked very well, and I've published the recipe in two other books. See this recipe at my website, NutritionCare.net, if your baby is failing with commercial formulas.

Since I am always asked, I will mention one last approach many parents swear by, but health professionals sternly admonish, and that is using raw milk to make formulas for babies. Proponents of raw cow's milk claim many health benefits from it, as well as claiming detrimental effects from pasteurized, homogenized milk from grain-fed (rather than grass-fed) cows. They also rightly point out that raw milk contains enzymes and probiotic activity that help protein digestion; these are destroyed by pasteurization. Pasteurization and homogenization alter the configuration of the protein and fats in milk, so that they are harder still to digest. Proponents submit that these reconfigured molecules trigger more allergy and inflammation, too. While this may be true, it's obviously not a measure anyone on your health care team will be willing to condone. Tainted milk has been fingered for causing tuberculosis for over a century, but recent genomic studies on the bacteria strains involved have cast doubt on this. If you would like more information about raw milk, visit the Weston Price Foundation on the web or see raw-milk-facts.com. Be aware that milk quality and safety are affected by what animals are fed, how and where they are raised, and how milk is collected, stored, and transported. If you would like to explore this option for your family, thoroughly screen your milk producer for reputation, farming practices, cleanliness, and safety record.

One other part of the colic story that deserves mention is gas. Switching formulas, feeding strategies, or your own diet if you are nursing is a quick fix for this most of the time. Besides struggling to digest a formula that doesn't sit well, gas in infants can also be triggered simply by swallowing too much air while feeding. If your baby has gas with normal stools, no skin changes, and a good growth pattern, this may be more likely. You can:

- Burp your baby more frequently during feeding, after every 2 or 3 ounces or between breasts.

- If you are breast-feeding, minimize foods that trigger gas for you (onions? broccoli? cabbage?). If this also means dairy foods, remove the dairy and add back ample calcium, minerals, fat, and protein sources such as kale soup, beef stew with tomatoes and vegetables, fermented soy foods such as tempeh and miso soup, green beans, carrot juice, eggs, enriched almond milk, or spoonfuls of sesame tahini in smoothies and oatmeal.

- Notice whether the usual suspects that you eat bother your baby: Chocolate, caffeine, dairy foods, citrus foods, and tomatoes often set off a nursing baby when Mom eats them.

- Many medications end up in mother's milk. Scrutinize this possibility before nursing while on a medication.

- Some babies have a disorganized "suck-swallow-breathe" (SSB) sequence that makes feeding inefficient, less effective, or lets in too much air. Babies born earlier than thirty-six weeks can be especially prone to this, but so can term infants who have special needs. Check with a lactation consultant, through your pediatrician or hospital, to assure that your baby is latching onto your breast in a way that allows efficient feeding. Your local Early Intervention Program provider or La Leche League (check the index for websites that can direct you to this) may have free resources that permit a consultant to visit you and your baby in your home to assist you.

What about medications or drops for gas? These are items such as simethicone drops, which are sold under dozens of over-the-counter brand names (for example, Mylicon) for all age groups, including infants. They may help as a short-term solution but don't solve the problem. If your baby has gas so hard and persisting as to need a medication for it indefinitely, look for the cause and treat that instead. Doing so may help your baby grow, sleep, eat, and play more contentedly anyway. Here's why a simethicone product such as infant Mylicon drops is not a good long-term tool (more than two weeks):

- Mylicon's manufacturer (Merck) issued a recall for it in late 2008, owing to "concerns for metal fragments generated during the manufacturing process." If your household contains Mylicon drops from that time, throw them out.

- Simethicone does not reduce gas, or prevent it from forming in the intestine. It exerts a chemical action that makes small gas bubbles combine into larger ones, so that they are easier and quicker to burp or, um, expel out the other end. This chemical is a foaming agent also used in industrial processes.

- Many simethicone products including infant Mylicon drops contain artificial colors, sugars, and/or artificial flavors, which many infants and older children don't tolerate.

- As long ago as 1994, a study in *Pediatrics* showed simethicone to be *less* effective than placebo in reducing colic; 22 percent of subjects had worsened gas symptoms while using this agent.

- A 1999 study in the *British Medical Journal* compared several drugs, diets, herbs, and behavioral measures for colic. The most successful treatment was replacing ordinary cow's milk formula (for example, Enfamil, Similac) with hypoallergenic formula (Nutramigen, Alimentum). Notably, reducing lactose in formula had no beneficial effect.

- In the same study, herbal blends scored higher than simethicone in reducing colic. See Chapter 2 for a discussion of those helpful herbs and safely using them in infants.

- Many drugs interfere with how foods and nutrients are absorbed. While simethicone does not appear to block any nutrients for absorption in the intestine, using it long-term can mask other problems that may be interfering with good absorption.

What about constipation? Babies who are formula fed experience this more often, and tend to have fewer, firmer stools than breast-fed infants overall. Introducing solids too early or too quickly can constipate babies also. When your baby can't move her bowels at least every two days, this is fine as long as she is growing, sleeping, cooing, exploring, and doing happy baby things. If there are signs of distress, then intervene; some may go for several days with no bowel movement. Not good, especially if this is routine. Some babies find soy formula more constipating. This may be due to difficulty digesting that protein source, or due to the additional iron in it. Since soy interferes with iron absorption, infant formulas made with soy protein have higher iron content. Here are nutrition-focused options to ease constipation for your baby:

- Try the goat milk infant formula recipe on page 251, if you have already found that your baby can't manage breast milk or regular infant formula.

- Try the semi-elemental formulas (Nutramigen or Alimen-tum), if your baby uses cow's milk or soy formula. If your baby is breast-fed and having more than three runny, liquid stools daily, consider the semi-elemental formulas as well.

- Introduce pureed stewed prunes or a few ounces of prune juice daily.

- Add ¼ cup Epsom salts to your baby's bath to enrich magnesium and sulfur, which will be absorbed through the skin. It's okay if a slurp or two is swallowed, but don't feed this orally or let your baby drink ounces of it.

- Herbs such as licorice and fennel have been safely used in babies to ease constipation. Talk to a licensed naturopathic doctor on how to use this option safely. If you don't know one, check Naturopathic.org on the web for the American Association of Naturopathic Doctors.

Seizures

Seizure events in a baby are one of the most frightening things a parent can experience. It can be difficult to know what is going on, and whether it is really a concern. What do seizures look like? This is one of the tricky parts. Not all seizures are dramatic events that rock a baby's entire body. They can be quite subtle: A startling reflex for no reason, lip smacking or head dropping, eyes fluttering or lilting upward or sideways, a vacant stare in which you can't get your baby's attention that happens at random times—these are worth mentioning to your doctor, as are random rocking or shaking movements that your baby can't stop, even if you hold him. Babies may also show a start, limb twitch, or jerking movements as they fall asleep, and this can be entirely normal. Your pediatrician may help you sort out which symptoms need more investigating.

If indeed your baby is having seizures, there are a few items to review on the nutrition checklist. I encourage this wherever possible, alongside the neurology consult process. In some cases, seizures may be relieved by these measures.

- Rule out bowel infections, and treat them. Certain products of gut microbe metabolism can trigger seizures. Consider antifungal medication, antibiotics if indicated by stool culture, and high-potency probiotics to quickly restore safe and healthy bifidobacteria and lactobacillus strains mentioned earlier in this chapter. Use a lab that extensively cultures and identifies specific strains for clostridia, candida, klebsiella, other fungal and bacterial species, and beneficial flora strains as well. Microbes excrete their own organic acids and toxins, which can cross the baby's delicate, permeable blood-brain barrier. Their effects on the infant brain are not well studied, but they have been shown to worsen features of autism in older children. In research using mice, brain tissue has been shown to react with seizures to proprionic acid, which is made by clostridia in the human gut. I have also witnessed improvement in seizures in children treated for intestinal candidiasis with an antifungal medication such as Diflucan.

- For a newborn, rule out bilirubin neurotoxicity, kernicterus, and infant jaundice. Bilirubin is made by the liver when breaking down old red blood cells, and it is a normal component of bile. It is eliminated in stool. Bilirubin will damage the baby's brain if it gets too high. Babies with too much bilirubin look jaundiced. If you think your baby's skin looks too yellow or orange, inform your doctor right away. Jaundice occurs often in babies and is not necessarily damaging, but it can progress to kernicterus, which is the medical term for brain-damaging neurotoxicity from bilirubin. Warning signs are a high-pitched cry, arching back, lethargy and difficulty arousing the baby, and unusual floppiness, low tone, or stiff tone. Some of these signs can be confused with seizures. In either case, they are serious signs that need immediate attention. Known causes of kernicterus include some vaccines and vaccine ingredients. Some published recommendations encourage avoidance of vaccines and vitamin K at birth, to prevent kernicterus (see *Developmental Medicine and Child Neurology*, November 2008).

- Trial an elemental, free amino acid protein source formula such as Elecare or infant Neocate. This will prevent damage to brain tissue from diet-sourced protein molecules or large protein fragments. Like bilirubin, these may cross into the brain in young infants.

- Discuss using pyridoxine (vitamin B6) and magnesium, two nutrients that help nerve impulse transmission in the brain. Dosage and administration should be determined by your neurologist, who may choose to give this orally, through a feeding tube, or through an IV. These nutrients may work even in circumstances where medications have failed to control seizures. Both large and ordinary doses of pyridoxine have been effective, based on published reports. Pyridoxine needs magnesium to work properly in cells, so including this in the protocol is prudent. It is believed that pyridoxine-dependent seizure disorders are genetically determined. If your baby did not respond to pyridoxine early on, she may when she is a bit older, so some recommendations suggest revisiting this tool after a few months on prescription anti-convulsant therapy.

Read any vaccine package insert, and you will see that seizures are a known possible side effect of an immunization. Read reports in the Vaccine Adverse Event Reporting System (previously inaccessible but made available through the Freedom of Information Act), and you will see that seizures are repeatedly documented by medical personnel as part of an adverse reaction to vaccinations. If your baby has shown signs of kernicterus, jaundice, or seizure activity, proceeding very cautiously with vaccinations is prudent at any age, but especially in infancy when the blood-brain barrier is more permeable and the brain itself, more vulnerable. Parents have the right to defer, reschedule, or refuse vaccinations in most states. Pediatricians are under blanket protections from federal law passed in the 1980s that frees them (and vaccine manufacturers) from any liability should a vaccine trigger seizures, other damage, or even death in your baby. This freedom certainly helps your pediatrician remain confident in giving vaccines; she suffers no consequence when a baby is injured by the shots she's administered. You and your child will, so take pains to educate yourself on safest strategies if your baby has already experienced problems mentioned here.

Of course, this will not be a welcome conversation to most pediatric MD providers; hostile press already exists on doctors who "fire" parents who won't vaccinate. As I said at the start of this chapter, trust your instincts; I have met hundreds of parents who regret that they did not. If your provider is combative or uncooperative, seek out a new provider who will support you in your journey to have a healthy, safe, happy child. Visit AskDrSears .com for tips on working with pediatricians who can support your concerns. Check Chapter 3 to review nutrition-focused tools that bolster a child's immune function if you are deferring vaccines, so you can minimize infections and illness. See the resources section for materials on vaccine safety. For more information on nutrition strategies in children over age one year who have seizures, as well as information on introducing solids, feeding, and growth for older babies and toddlers, see Chapter 4.

Chapter Two

Solutions for Sleep with Special-Needs Kids

When I was a new parent, I noticed a stark dividing line between the relaxed parents versus the anxious ones, the energetic versus the exhausted, the cheerful versus the struggling. The babies picked up on their parents' state, too. There were the contented cherubs, and the ones who seemed to note the stress filtering down to them. My hunch then was that this had a lot to do with sleep, and much research backs this up. Parents often feel ashamed or embarrassed by a child's inability to sleep well. It might seem that getting our babies to sleep is the first parenting task we are supposed to master. If we fail at that, then what? An unexpected shock in my own transition from pregnancy to new mom was having the freedom to sleep all night suddenly vanish. The unending battle to help our baby sleep left us frayed and depleted for months and beyond. This is no picnic for babies either, as sleeplessness can impact their growth, elevate stress chemistry, and defeat immune function. I didn't know then about many of the sleep-supporting, nutrition-focused tools that are easy for babies and parents to try.

How much wakefulness is too much for a newborn? Some guidelines follow below, but babies with special needs may have a harder time sleeping than entirely typical ones. Two or even three daily naps would be typical for a young infant. My own son often stayed awake all day in his first three months, looking woeful and haggard, in defiance of what all the baby books and doctors said, never napping despite our best efforts and routines. His nighttime sleep was like a sputtering lawn mower engine: It occurred in fits and starts, needed a lot of cajoling to get started, and was peppered with nerve-searing shrieks when it stopped (can you tell I need a new mower?).

Like hundreds of other little ones I've met, my baby had a litany of concerns around feeding, growth, and digestion. Address these, and your baby or child will likely sleep better. Who can sleep when they're hungry, have a stomachache or pants filled with stinging, wet stool, or feel gastrointestinal pain? How can you fall asleep if your brain doesn't make the right chemistry to tell it to do that? There is nothing to gain from leaving a baby to cry it out in these circumstances. When a baby doesn't fall asleep within a few days of trying on his own, then there is quite possibly an underlying physical reason. So if you've tried leaving your baby to cry herself to sleep, and it hasn't worked after more than a week, it is time to look for what else may be making her miserable. For many special-needs kids, this can be an even tougher nut to crack. Many parents I meet in practice have wakeful and wandering ten- or twelve-year-old children who have never had a normal sleep pattern in their entire lives. If this is you, take heart; tricks here may help everyone get a good rest yet.

Sleep deprivation and insomnia are serious for babies, kids, and their parents. We need to sleep deeply and without interruption to literally regenerate new tissue, and repair damaged tissue throughout the body. Certain phases of sleep are the only time when neurons in the cerebral cortex can regenerate. Other phases of sleep permit new synaptic connections to grow and form in the brain. Ages zero to three are the period of the most explosive growth in the brain, so you can see why babies and toddlers need to sleep a lot. In sleep-deprived test subjects, areas of the brain normally active for processing language showed no activity. They also showed less activity in the frontal lobe, which is where we generate imaginative words, ideas, and creative thinking. The test subjects used more monotonic speech, slower speech, and had more trouble forming sentences. Interesting to note, then, that up to 70 percent of children with autism spectrum disorders struggle with insomnia! Imagine how their lives might change if this could be resolved. It has also been found that rapid eye movement (REM) sleep is needed to lock in newly learned skills. Much research shows how crucial good sleep is to learning. If your special-needs child is struggling with her sleep pattern, this is one problem you can improve with nutrition-focused tools.

We all know that poor sleep impacts more than just the brain, in people of all ages. Not sleeping enough lowers white blood cell count, a critical line of defense against infection, and alters our hormonal response to stress. Baby's poor sleep pattern correlates with postnatal depression in moms—and babies born to moms with depression tend to have more chaotic sleep patterns. So put sleep high on your priority to-do list. There is no virtue in wading through months of poor sleep with a baby, toddler, or older child, and it can harm your child's behavior, growth, learning, and development, too. Before you presume that a child's poor sleep pattern is all about manipulation (as my pediatrician told me when my son was just four weeks old), or an unalterable by-product of a special-needs diagnosis, remember that children, too, need sleep as much as you if not more, and would probably welcome it just as much. Use these safe techniques and see what works for you. Individuals vary; while taurine may relax Dad nicely, it may do nothing for junior, who needs melatonin and some chamomile. Don't assume everyone in the household will respond to each potential tool the same way.

Follow all the usual sleep hygiene advice. Obviously, implement those nap and bedtime routines. Let older siblings help with the easy parts, such as getting baby's PJs and bed ready, looking through a baby book with bedtime feeding, or feeding baby if she is not at the breast. This is winding-down family time. The same goes for toddlers and school-age children: Routines matter. Parents need to team up on placing that line in the sand around their own space in the evening. Even with high-needs children, the point comes where Mom and Dad get their space and service has ended for the night, barring exceptional situations and requirements such as administering medications or checking tube feed pumps.

Make sure foods are well tolerated. Children with special needs such as autism, Down's syndrome, diabetes, ADHD, or Crohn's disease are more likely to have inflammation triggered by food proteins. This will mean more problems with growth, feeding, digesting, and absorbing food. Children with inflammation from foods may have reflux, constipation and/or diarrhea, and stomachaches more often, which can make sleeping a lot harder. If your child sleeps in a yoga position called the "child pose," that is, facedown with knees to chest, upright only, or with abdomen jackknifed over a pillow or mattress, you need to rule out concerns such as fecal impactions, reflux, or bowel infections. Candida (fungal species or yeast), clostridia or *Helicobacter pylori* (types of bacteria), or other disruptive bowel pathogens can flourish happily in the intestine without causing frank illness or fever, but they may cause pain, inflammation, stooling problems, picky appetites, or even ulcers. These are easy to rule out. See the resources section to learn how.

Your doctor may have checked your child for food allergies already. A food allergy is a swift immune reaction to a food, mediated by a protein we make called Immunoglobulin E (IgE). Symptoms of a food allergy are plain: hives; vomiting; swelling in the throat, lips, or eyes; tingling of the lips, tongue, or throat; or sudden onset of stomach pain. Obviously, if your child has shown these signs, you know it already. You are likely avoiding that trigger food, have antihistamine medicines handy, or use an EpiPen in emergencies. Children with allergies will have high circulating levels of IgE, either in total and/or to a particular food. Blood and skin prick tests can diagnose this, along with signs and symptoms.

More insidious but still problematic, especially for infants and children, are food *sensitivities*. In 1984, the American Academy of Allergy and Immunology defined these as "an immunologic reaction to a food, often delayed, that may not involve IgE antibody, but may involve IgG." This was more than thirty-five years ago, so it still puzzles me that I have met only one or two pediatric physicians over my years in practice who acknowledge, much less understand, food sensitivities. A number of researchers have documented that IgG-mediated food sensitivities can impair growth in children, cause loose, wet stool, trigger stomachaches, or worsen reflux. IgG-mediated reactions occur more slowly and insidiously than IgE reactions. Symptoms showing that these are active in your child are irritability that waxes and wanes for no apparent reason, gray circles under the eyes, frequent runny nose or mucus in the throat, asthma, weak appetite, a narrow appetite (will only eat a few foods), a growth pattern that isn't quite as strong as expected or even frank growth regression, reflux, sensory integration problems, or an irritable mixed stool pattern. Paradoxically, children often crave and prefer foods that trigger IgG reactions.

In infants, IgG-mediated milk protein sensitivity is a classic cause of colic. As mentioned in Chapter 1, a 1998 review in the *British Medical Journal* (ancient history in terms of published research) compared several treatments for colic in infants. The most common tool—simethicone (Mylicon) drops—was the least effective. The most effective remedy was switching cow's milk protein–based formulas, such as Similac or Enfamil, to easier-to-digest formulas, such as Nutramigen, Alimentum, Neocate Infant, or Carnation Good Start. Switching to soy protein formulas was not very effective, though it may help some infants; my experience in practice mirrors what this study found, which is that soy protein is intolerable to babies almost as often as cow's milk protein is.

Milk protein (regardless of which type of milk it's from) is also called casein. Cow casein is very different from human casein. It is harder to digest. In pasteurization, it undergoes molecular changes that make it even harder still to digest. About half of all babies just can't do it. Refer back to Chapter 1 for instructions on how to switch your baby's formula if she is struggling with crying and colic instead of sleeping.

It's easy to diagnose protein intolerance in an infant under six months old, because infants at this age only eat one major protein source—your casein from breast milk, cow casein in formula, or soy protein in formula. No blood tests are needed to ascertain this. Eliminate the problem protein, and your baby will sleep better immediately. Replace irritating, inflammatory formula with something easier to digest and absorb. See Chapter 1 for more detail on infant feeding.

Youngsters eating several food proteins may need some testing to sort out what is what. If the child's diet includes only a few proteins, it can be easy to start by eliminating the major suspects; beneficial effects on sleep should appear in a week or two. If we are talking about an older child, an ELISA IgG food antibody panel can check dozens of foods using a simple blood spot test that requires only five drops of blood from your child's finger or toe. These have been found in clinical trials to be as or more reliable than elimination diets in discerning inflammatory foods. ELISA IgG testing is suitable for children over age two or three; it is not informative for children under age eighteen months. False positives may abound on this test in children under two years old, in my experience. Lastly, don't make the very common error of removing every single food that shows any reactivity on this panel. This leaves children on impossibly restricted, inadequate diets. Pick the top three or four biggest offenders, or only those that are the highest reactivity (identified as 3+ or 4+ on the panel), and rotate the rest. Add in gut-replenishing tools such as probiotics, liposomal glutathione, treatment for bowel infections if they are active, and free amino acids. Debate and confusion abound about whether this test is useful, and how to interpret it. Long and short, yes, it is useful and accurate enough to be a helpful tool in my practice, as long as it is used correctly. For more detail on this, see my previous book, *Special-Needs Kids Eat Right*, published in 2009.

Know what is typical for your baby or child's age, stage, and special-needs diagnosis. Young infants go through a complete sleep cycle in about an hour and can wake many times during the night. By age four months, they should be able to fall asleep without much fanfare and regularly enjoy a six-to-eight-hour stretch of sleep. Infants with special needs may not be able to do that. Make sure nutrition problems are not interfering; see above about ruling out inflammatory foods, reflux, or bowel infections. School-age children need between nine and twelve hours of sleep a night. Kids should be able to fall asleep in about fifteen to thirty minutes, and stay asleep. They should be able to wake up pretty easily in the morning, and not need a lot of cajoling to get out of bed. Here is a nutrition checklist to run through before you try that Ferber method of letting your child cry himself to sleep or get upset that your eight-year-old is at your bedside again at 1:15 a.m., tapping you on the shoulder just as you've dropped off.

- Are they getting enough total calories? Babies, toddlers, and even older children will wake at night if they are not eating enough total calories on a regular basis. See *Special-Needs Kids Eat Right* for detailed information on the calories that kids need.

- Infants and toddlers need roughly 45–50 calories for every pound, every day.

- Underweight infants may need double this amount. If your baby is low weight, below the 10th percentile in weight for age after starting near the middle of the chart, or born at a low weight for gestational age, ask your pediatrician for a nutrition care referral. A registered dietitian will calculate how much food or formula your baby needs each day to start growing more typically (pediatricians don't do this, dietitians do). Or contact me through NutritionCare.net for a consult.

- A child's daily calorie needs per pound generally drop a bit around age four, then again toward age seven, and again during puberty. Parents of special-needs children who are underweight or overweight can get exact guidance on this from a registered dietitian, or contact me through NutritionCare .net for more help.

- Can they digest and absorb formula, breast milk, or foods comfortably? Inflammation from foods, diminished enzyme output in the GI tract, or untreated bowel infections may interfere enough to trigger pain, reflux, gas, or other discomforts that wake your child up and make him miserable.

- If you are using a pump and tube feeding during the night, make sure the food or formula is entirely appropriate. Rule out inflammatory proteins with ELISA IgG if you've already done an IgE allergy panel that was negative.

- Rule out bowel infections with a stool microbiology panel from a lab such as Doctor's Data. This lab will differentiate and culture healthy bowel bacteria strains, to show whether or not your child's intestine hosts beneficial species such as lactobacillus and bifidobacteria strains. Doctor's Data will also culture and differentiate various candida species and detrimental bacteria that tend to trigger diarrhea, such as klebsiella or campylobacter species. Your pediatrician can help screen for clostridia, another infamous trigger for malabsorption and diarrhea.

• If mucus buildup and vomiting are regular challenges for your tube-fed youngster, consider adding a mucus-specific enzyme such as Mucostop to the feeding. Review the foods for tolerance or inflammation, and review the possibility of bowel infections. Both these problems may exacerbate mucus.

How to rule out reflux. Many parents are advised to give an infant or young child a reflux medication, when there is too much spit-up, colic, or gas. These can aid sleep if reflux is worse at night, when lying down. But using these for longer than a week or two comes with a price. Over time, these medications may alter the pH of the entire digestive tract, shifting it away from the pH needed for optimal digestion and beneficial gut microbes that grow in the intestine. Losing beneficial gut microbes means disruptive ones move in, and this means more digestive problems, more inflammatory conditions, more stooling problems, and even more reflux. My own observation in practice is that babies who use reflux medications throughout their first year have more digestion, feeding, growth, and sensory processing problems by the time they are three or four years old than babies who never used this medication or used it very little. Before you use medications such as Prevacid for reflux, try a few simple troubleshoots at home first:

- Give your child a calcium carbonate supplement (such as TUMS) at bedtime. This is especially indicated for the child who can only sleep upright, or "postures" often (for example, pulls knees, pillows, coffee table, or other firm object to press against the abdomen) in order to sleep. Little ones who cannot use a calcium carbonate chewable can try a liquid calcium carbonate supplement in a little soft food or evening feeding. About 200 milligrams of calcium are enough for this test, and you can check with your pediatrician to be sure. If your baby or child sleeps better, then she may have an overly acidic stomach that burns the esophagus, or a mechanical issue that permits the valve at the end of the esophagus to open too freely (discuss these possibilities with your doctor). Your child may sleep better with her head slightly elevated above the stomach also.

- If calcium carbonate worsens the problem and your child has more discomfort, give ½ teaspoon plain cider vinegar in a bit of lemonade, apple juice, or water. This will acidify rather than buffer the stomach. Reflux can occur when the stomach is not acid *enough*. This is because the stomach needs to be very acidic in order to initiate digestion. Food entering the stomach is immediately worked on by the acid there. This also signals the pylorus to open (the valve where your stomach ends and small intestine begins) and lets the stomach's highly acid contents proceed into the small intestine, where the acidity further stimulates the release of enzymes and hormones that let digestion progress. A stomach that is too buffered is a stomach where food may sit for hours, which makes ample opportunity for refluxing. If your child is not sick, has no fever, and frequently vomits undigested food from a meal eaten eight to ten hours before, it is likely that the acidity of her stomach is too weak. Even though in this case the stomach is not acid enough to properly initiate digestion, it is still acid enough to irritate the esophagus, and it will. If a bit of vinegar (which is mildly acid) soothes your child, you can use it to gently acidify your child's stomach just enough to aid digestion normally. Only use it when the need is obvious, based on your child's signs, complaints, or symptoms.

If these tools are inconclusive or unsuccessful, talk to your pediatrician about a pH probe test for your child. This will ascertain precisely what the pH of your child's stomach is and how often he actually refluxes. It will become clear if a medication is warranted. If it is, have a plan for how long you will use it and how you will wean off it. See Chapter 4 for more detail on further troubleshoots for bowel infections and other GI problems.

Use a warm bath to induce relaxation. Add Epsom salts (magnesium sulfate), baking soda, and a drop of lavender essential oil to your child's nightly bath. A ten- or fifteen-minute bath suffices to let the minerals in the salts be absorbed. Epsom salts contain magnesium, a mineral needed for calm and smooth nerve transmission, and sulfur, an element needed for liver and digestive enzymes, for managing inflammatory responses plus many structural proteins in the body. Sulfur is needed to run several metabolic processes that permit safe excretion of phenols, additives, colorings, heavy metals, and even medications. Both the magnesium and sulfate in Epsom salts are well absorbed through skin.

These are typically calming, but some children have an antagonistic reaction and will be agitated or more active and awake rather than relaxed and sleepy. Some research shows that persons with autism are depleted of sulfur, and while they need to replenish this critical element, doing so too quickly may trigger a run of sorts on the detoxification pathways dependent on it. This may mean your child is suddenly working overtime to eliminate toxins that have been backed up because of low sulfur supply. If you note an agitated response, perhaps this is the case; use a very small amount of Epsom salts (a spoonful or two) and slowly work up as tolerated. Restoring normal sulfation chemistry will be beneficial in the long term.

Note: Medications may be metabolized more efficiently when Epsom salts are used, which may mean more medicine actually gets to the bloodstream even when the dose stays the same. Some children I have worked with were able to lower dosages of medications (especially psychiatric medications) after replenishing sulfur with Epsom salts. Be sure to watch for changes in your child's response to a medication if you use Epsom salts. Let your doctor know about it. Your child may be able to use less medication, too. Any sudden response after using Epsom salts is an indicator that sulfur chemistry was probably depleted. Sulfur is not an easy element to absorb from the gut. Continue with the baths, but lower the amount of Epsom salts you use, until a calm and happy medium is found.

Try essential oils that may induce sleep. Add an essential oil such as lavender for an extra-relaxing effect. One to four drops of an essential oil will be ample for a tub; do not use essential oils directly on skin. Besides soothing lavender, try a drop or two of sandalwood or frankincense in a warm bath or in a massage oil. These have compounds in them called sesquiterpenes that may act on the pineal gland, a tiny structure in the brain responsible for releasing melatonin. Melatonin is a hormone that makes us fall asleep (babies normally make lots of melatonin, while kids hitting puberty make less). Other calming effects may be had with essential oils of melissa, red cedar, ylang-ylang, or clary sage. Avoid stimulating oils or fragrances in shampoos, lotions, or soaps used at bedtime, such as peppermint, spearmint, orange, citrus, lemongrass, tea tree, jasmine, patchouli, or eucalyptus. Try one oil at a time, one drop at a time, when using with small children. Avoid those you know are triggering for inflammation in other forms—that is, if your child sneezes from sniffing geraniums or gets red and itchy after drinking citrus juices, these are plant families to avoid when considering drops of their essential oils in the tub.

- For a baby tub (countertop size), add ¼ cup Epsom salts, ¼ cup baking soda, and 1 drop lavender or essential oil of your choice.

- For a toddler in a regular tub, add ½ cup salts, ½ cup baking soda, and 2–3 drops lavender.

- For big kids (60 pounds or more), up to a cup of Epsom salts is okay, plus ½ cup baking soda and 4 drops lavender.

- For tired moms and dads, give yourself the same care before you go to bed if you have time. Bathe in 2 cups Epsom salts, 1 cup baking soda, and any relaxing essential oil you like.

Support melatonin production. The essential amino acid trypto-phan is needed to make melatonin. If you don't have enough tryp-tophan around, melatonin will be hard to make. You can be short on tryptophan if you don't eat enough total protein, or if you don't digest protein very well. I meet many kids in practice with *both* problems, so no wonder they can't sleep well.

It works like this: There are about twenty-two amino acids known. About eight of these, including tryptophan, are "essential" to human life—that is, we must eat them to live. The remaining fourteen or so amino acids can be manufactured in our own cells, by rearranging the essential ones. Amino acids are the building blocks of protein; if a protein is a strand of pearls, each pearl is an amino acid. When we digest protein, we liberate those individ-ual pearls. They are then absorbed from the gut and distributed bodywide, to be reassembled into tissue, structures, hormones, neurotransmitters, enzymes, and so forth.

One problem I frequently see in young children in my practice is that they may not extract these aminos very well from the pro-tein in their diets. They don't release the individual pearls from the necklace, either because of a digestive insufficiency or a gut wall that lets oversize molecules across when it shouldn't. This lets protein enter the bloodstream as poorly digested peptides— that is, like small strands of a pearl necklace rather than individual pearls. These pearl strands have limited value in the machinery that makes stuff such as melatonin. The machinery needs indi-vidual pearls, not chunks of pearls stuck together. This seems to leave kids bereft of the building blocks they need to make the right balance of neurotransmitters or hormones. Nutritional paths can be leveraged to help assure that those pearls of tryptophan are available to the brain toward evening or bedtime.

- Include tryptophan-rich foods at the end of the day, if your child can tolerate them: turkey, chicken, beef, brown rice, eggs, cheese, nuts, lentils, and milk.

- Milk and dairy foods are rich in tryptophan. But chances are if you have a little one who sleeps poorly, milk and dairy foods may be part of the problem. Be sure you rule this out. Use an ELISA IgG test, or check signs and symptoms (Chapter 4) that indicate that dairy protein is not being assimilated normally.

- Children with autism may also consider a urine casomorphin peptide test. If milk protein (casein) is poorly digested, it can show up in urine as a peptide called casomorphin. Persons with autism have been shown to have elevated diet-sourced peptides such as casomorphin in urine as much as 80 percent of the time. This peptide has documented activity at endorphin and morphine receptors in the brain. Children absorbing casomorphin into brain tissue often have disrupted sleep patterns. They tend to wake between midnight and 3 a.m., often talking, laughing, or playing. Other signs of high urine peptides are constipation, a rigid eating pattern, and aphasia. Use the urine test to rule this out. If it's positive, you will need to withdraw casein and probably gluten as well, since both form similar opiate-like peptides. See *Special-Needs Kids Eat Right* for details on this and how to safely feed your child on a gluten-free, casein-free (GFCF) diet.

- Tryptophan enters the brain more quickly when eaten with carbs. So if your child drinks milk at bedtime, give it with a small treat such as toast and jam, applesauce, half a warm scone, or a warm slice of pumpkin or zucchini bread. If it's turkey you're offering, warm a slice or two and give with cranberry jelly or chutney, gravy, cooked beets, or warm potato (great if these are leftovers and you aren't cooking a second dinner).

- If milk and dairy foods are problematic, try egg and toast, beef chili and rice, a small serving of lentil soup (I like Amy's brand because it's ready-to-heat and organic), or a favorite nut butter or sesame butter (tahini) on toast.

- All of these bedtime snack and dinner ideas can be modified to be gluten-, dairy-, soy-, or egg-free. See the resources section for allergy-free meal planning resources.

If high-tryptophan foods toward evening aren't cutting it and your child is still wakeful, this may indicate that the tryptophan is not getting where it needs to go. Especially if your child has any signs of trouble with bowel movements, either too firm and too few (less than one per day) or too loose and too many, it's possible that those tryptophan "pearls" aren't coming off the necklace of dietary protein. I would further suspect this if your child has trouble with anxiety, depressed affect (even young children can be depressed), or aggression, because tryptophan is also needed to make serotonin.

The good news is you can easily enrich this pathway with a supplement. For children age five or 60 pounds and up, you can try this tool for better sleep. Tryptophan is available as a supplement itself, or in another form called 5-hydroxytryptophan (5-HTP), which is two metabolic steps away from melatonin. The neurotransmitter in between? Serotonin. Serotonin regulates mood, appetite, and aggression. Start with a 25-milligram dose near bedtime with a carbohydrate snack such as applesauce, toast with jam, or even a cookie (do not give with milk, soy milk, or protein foods for this test). You can open a capsule and stir it into applesauce, spread it on toast hidden in jam or nut butter, or plop it into a bedtime fruit smoothie. Go up in 25-milligram increments every two or three nights, but do not give more than the amount necessary to improve sleep. Do not give adult dosages of 5-HTP to a child. Your child may only need this tool for a few weeks, then their own chemistry may be balanced enough to carry on without the supplement. Smaller children will probably do well taking 25–50 milligrams; older school-age children or teens may stop at 100 milligrams. Amino acids are in and out of the body quickly. If your child has an antagonistic reaction, that is, is wakeful and agitated, this should pass within twenty-four hours, or even less. *Children using SSRIs or any medication that may impact serotonin level should not use 5-hydroxytryptophan without medical supervision. Check with your prescriber first.*

Caution! Small children under 60 pounds should not be given any serotonin boosters without medical supervision, whether they are pharmaceutical or nutritional. Serotonin can be toxic to the nervous system if it gets too high, and this can be caused by medications as well as nutrition tools. Don't combine pharmaceuticals such as SSRIs (Paxil, Zolofit, Prozac, etc.) with nutritional supplements such as tryptophan, 5-HTP, or Saint John's wort. These *all* boost serotonin. Ask your psychiatric MD prescriber for more information if you'd like to consider using these tools in smaller children. Symptoms of serotonin toxicity are rapid heart rate, dilated pupils, extreme drowsiness, low blood pressure, perspiration, feeling dizzy or "drunk," overreactive reflexes, or a hypervigilant or agitated affect. If you note these symptoms after giving a supplement such as tryptophan, 5-HTP, or a medication, call your health care provider immediately, or go to the emergency room if they worsen. You should also call your doctor if this occurs after giving a prescription psychiatric medication. These can be dangerous if your child does not tolerate them as expected.

Use melatonin itself. As mentioned earlier, melatonin is not a medication, but a hormone we make ourselves to signal the brain into sleep. I have not used melatonin in children younger than eighteen months. Is it safe for infants? Probably, but this is a question to review with your pediatrician. Infants make a lot of melatonin naturally; if they aren't sleeping, it may be quite depleted, a state that is possibly detrimental for them. Some research suggests that melatonin may be lifesaving when it comes to SIDS: Infants who die from SIDS have very low levels of melatonin in their brains. Because melatonin is a powerful antioxidant, there is speculation that it may play a role in preventing the severe, life-threatening oxidative stress that occurs with SIDS. Discuss giving your baby melatonin with your health care professional.

If your infant is persisting in a stressful, screaming pattern at night instead of sleeping, melatonin may be useful, but ask your pediatrician about dosing first. Prolonged screaming is not healthy for infants. It is extremely costly for them, in terms of energy balance. Young infants need more than twice the calories per pound that a school-age child requires in order to maintain a normal growth pattern. When an infant is awake more than normal, or expending precious energy screaming night after night instead of sleeping, growth can suffer. This can, of course, also harm an infant's delicate emotional well-being and threaten normal attachment to his or her parent.

Young children should not need more than 1–2 milligrams of

melatonin per night. Start with a very low dose, and as always, inform your provider team before you start. Use the least amount to encourage sleep, and no more. Many preparations for melatonin are available that are suited to children, as drops, melting wafers, chewables, or sublingual sprays. These are given under the tongue and work fairly quickly; they don't need to pass through the stomach and small intestine to take effect. Some parents give melatonin thirty to sixty minutes before bedtime, to shorten the time it takes a child to actually drop off. Rules for using melatonin:

- Start with a quarter-milligram dose for young toddlers.

- Start with a half-milligram if your child is two years or older.

- Stop at the lowest effective dose. More is not necessarily better.

- Children with autism may need more. Still start at a low dose, and work up slowly.

- Older children (70 pounds or more) can start with a 1-milligram dose.

- Periodically try weaning your child off melatonin. He may no longer need it.

- An effective dose lets your child fall asleep in about thirty minutes or less, and stay asleep, most nights per week.

- Don't use melatonin preparations with other supplements in them. If there is a problem, you won't know which component is causing the trouble.

- Avoid melatonin preparations that include pyridoxine (vitamin B6). This vitamin can trigger wakefulness. Your child may do fine with extra B6 early in the day, but may struggle to sleep if it is given at night.

Children with autism, anxiety, depression, or other mood disorders may benefit from a higher dose of melatonin. If your doctor isn't sure on dosing, ask for a referral to someone who *is* sure. This may be a psychiatrist, a naturopathic doctor, or even a neurologist. A clinical trial that used melatonin in children with autism showed no side effects, other than good ones: There was a reduction in compulsive and ritualistic behaviors while the kids with autism used melatonin. Some of the children needed up to 6 milligrams of melatonin to reap benefits. All children are different, so start with the smallest appropriate dose and use only what is needed to elicit the benefit of sleep.

Enrich calming neurotransmitter pathways with other amino acids. While melatonin is a hormone we make from amino acids in the brain, individual amino acids themselves have different effects, from calming to stimulating. Amino acids are extracted from the protein we eat, and we make some of them ourselves as well. They quickly leave the body and cannot "build up," as a medication does. If an amino acid supplement is useful for your child, you should note its benefits within a week or less.

I do not usually use amino acids in my own practice in children under three or four years old. Infants and young children will probably be aided to sleep by other tools first, such as Epsom salts baths, essential oils, changed formula or foods, or herbs. If you still want to try amino acids for a child under four or so, supervision with a knowledgeable MD or ND (naturopathic doctor) provider is advisable. Though amino acid supplements have a better safety record than psychiatric medications, keeping your doctor in the loop is wise.

Balancing calming chemistry during the day can help children sleep at night, so you may want to work on that before dosing with amino acids at bedtime. To try calming amino acids at bedtime, start with only one at a time and use the lowest effective dose. Taurine, theanine, and gamma-aminobutyric acid (GABA) are soothing and calming. These have been used for children (and adults) with autism, obsessive-compulsive disorder (OCD), extreme reactivity, or anxiety. They are often used in the daytime to abate these features in children, and you may find they are more useful during daylight hours for your child. See Chapter 5 for more information on using these amino acid supplements. If you still want to try them at bedtime, stick to these suggestions for using amino acids:

- Start with low doses and only use the least effective dose. More may not be better.

- Periodically wean your child off an amino acid supplement. He may no longer need it. Resume the supplement only if it is clear that he does still need it.

- If your child uses medications for seizures, mood, depression, attention, or behavior, *always tell your prescriber before using amino acid supplements*. They may not mix with your child's medication, or may potentiate a medication's effects because they may target the same neurotransmitter pathways. This is especially true for medications treating seizures, mood, attention, or psychiatric concerns.

Taurine is an amino acid that is especially plentiful in meat and fish, and not surprisingly, it has been found to be low in people who eat vegan diets. It is nonessential, meaning we can manufacture it in our own bodies if need be. In humans, it is most abundant in brain, heart, and eye tissue. Taurine is an "inhibitory" amino acid, meaning it calms rather than excites nerve cell transmissions. It may have antiseizure effects; one thing taurine does is influence how potassium, sodium, and magnesium move in and out of cells. It tends to keep sodium out, and magnesium and potassium in, which may be helpful for those with seizures or tics. It may also protect against calcium rushing too quickly between nerve cells, an excitatory effect that may play a role in seizures. Perhaps this is why taurine is often suggested for children with autism, about a third of whom have seizure disorders and many of whom have anxiety.

Taurine is often used for calming or near bedtime, to aid sleep. Children weighing 40 pounds or more can be given a 50-milligram dose to start, and increase incrementally until an improvement is noted. There are no reports of toxicity from taurine in children. (Any food, supplement, or drug will have a dose at which it will either be toxic or trigger side effects; in taurine's case, this appears to be in the multigram range, and the only effects known are transient diarrhea or headache.) A dose of 200 milligrams is not unusual for a small child. Adults have been given up to 6 grams per day (that's 120 times more than 50 milligrams) in a trial reviewing its efficacy in congestive heart failure (results were positive). If your young child takes up to 600 milligrams with no benefit for sleep, check with an experienced provider before proceeding with higher doses. It may be that you are on the wrong track and need a different tool. Older children or children weighing more than 50 pounds can begin with 100 milligrams, and go up. Note: Blood and urine tests for taurine may not be very reliable, since reference ranges are wide and vary with age and weight. They also cannot directly measure the level of taurine in cells, where it is needed.

If you'd rather not use supplements such as 5-HTP or tryptophan, you can consider herbal supports for sleep. Many calming herb preparations are made for infants, toddlers, and children. Avoid stronger herbs that may be addicting or overly sedating, such as valerian (from which the drug Valium is derived) and alcohol tinctures. Look for glycerite tinctures instead. You can also make chamomile tea before bed with a small bit of honey, but this may have only a mild impact on a child with a deeply disrupted sleep pattern. Here are some examples of herbal products intended to help children sleep:

- WishGarden Herbs Quiet Time—glycerite tincture of passionflower, oat seed, and scullcap leaf.

- WishGarden Herbs Sleepy Nights—glycerite tincture of milky oat seed, passion flower leaf, linden flowers, scullcap leaf, and hawthorne berries.

- Mountain Rose Herbs Chamomile-Catnip Glycerite—tincture of chamomile, catnip, and lemon balm.

- Mountain Rose Herbs Oats Glycerite—tincture of milky green oat tops and vanilla flavoring.

- Individual tinctures of passion flower or scullcap leaf.

- Capsules of passion flower or scullcap, for older children who can swallow them.

Check with your prescriber first if your child takes a medication for sleep, mood, depression, or seizures, before using melatonin, herbs, tryptophan, or 5-HTP.

Make sure your child's diet is calmly absorbed. Other than helpful adjuncts such as supplements, herbs, teas, or essential oils in a bath, massage oil, or infuser at bedtime, make sure your child is eating and absorbing his diet normally. Children with special needs including autism, Down's syndrome, inflammatory conditions such as cystic fibrosis, bowel diseases, or ADHD and mood disorders may have gluten sensitivity more often than typical peers, according to emerging research. Antibodies made against gluten (the protein in wheat) move freely into anyplace in the body, including the brain, where other research shows they can trigger autoimmune reactions and damage to brain tissue. If this is true, you will want to know so your child's special needs are not confounded further by gluten exposure. This may impact growth, absorption, sleep, mood, and sensory processing.

What about children who fall asleep easily enough but can't stay asleep? Any of the tools mentioned so far may help, and you can use them during the night as well, with the caveat that the closer the hour is to morning, the sleepier your child may be when he is supposed to be waking up. A frequent finding in my practice for children with autism spectrum disorders or ADHD is wakefulness in the wee hours, say about 1 a.m. to 4 a.m. Parents will often describe a child who is alert, content, and ready to play;

some even report that the child is laughing and giggly. I've noted this often coincides with elevated exogenous opiates for the child, that is, the child's GI system makes too many opiate-like peptides out of ordinary food proteins—namely, wheat, dairy, or soy. This is the origin of the gluten-free, casein-free diet you may have heard about, which many families try for autism. It was later noted that soy protein can elicit essentially the same problem peptide as gluten and casein. A urine test can rule this out, as will a check for signs and symptoms. The following signs suggest a child is probably not digesting these proteins normally and may indeed be absorbing them mostly as opiate-like peptides that engage opiate receptors in the brain. Any one of these signs persisting for more than three or four weeks is suspect and would be on my radar, as a nutritionist, to troubleshoot and resolve:

- A tendency toward constipation or firm stools

- A history of constipation, impaction, or the need for laxatives

- Pupils seem more dilated than normal, especially after eating

- Rigidity in food choices (self-limited to dairy or wheat foods)

- A child past age one year who consumes most of his calories from milk and refuses solids

- A child who accepts only dairy as a protein source (yogurt, cheese, mac and cheese, milk, etc.)

- Aphasia (no expressive language)

- Delayed expressive language or problems with language processing/praxis

- Gobbles and devours food, or seeks out food with a vengeance, even if well fed

- Distinct behavior or mood change after eating—calmer, happier, silly, or laughing

- Distinct negative mood or reactive/violent when favorite or expected foods are denied or when hungry

Some persons with autism—adults and kids alike—exhibit extreme seeking behaviors around food, such that cabinets and refrigerator must be locked. Some will wake at dawn or predawn hours to rifle through cabinets, and can become agitated or even violent if interrupted or denied access to the food they seek. Children with ordinary hunger and calorie malnutrition may wake and cry at night, but they won't typically get up with an intense mission to bust open snack packages. They will also be able to return to sleep if given a brief nursing, feeding, or small something to eat. If your child is waking and seeking food nightly, screen for adequate total calories, then consider a urine polypeptide test to screen for diet-sourced opiate compounds. A pediatrician generally does not screen for low-calorie intakes. This is a dietitian's job, and requires a review of your child's food diary. Appropriate ranges for calorie intakes for children are explained in *Special-Needs Kids Eat Right*. If you aren't sure about reviewing this yourself, ask for a referral to a dietitian, who can review this for you. Some naturopathic doctors or holistically minded MDs may know about screening for urine polypeptides; others may not. See the resources section for a guideline on adequate total calories for kids, and how to order a urine polypeptide screening test.

For an infant, a child, or their families, chronically poor or inadequate sleep is devastating for overall health, learning, and well-being. Sleep is important, especially for maintaining a normal, functional stress response. Without it, immune function is quick to suffer. The next chapter outlines strategies to minimize infections—but these will work better in the context of reliable sleep for you and your child.

Chapter Three

Staying Healthy and Avoiding Infections

Can you imagine a winter in which you don't need to take the kids to the doctor for sick visits, you don't pick up any antibiotics for anyone in your house, and no one gets so much as a mild fever? Despite following recommended vaccine schedules and hygiene routines, kids get sick. In fact, they get *sicker* than they did before the days of using so many vaccines and antibiotics. The CDC reported a 20 percent increase in "unhealthy" days between 1993 and 2001, that is, sick days keeping parents and kids at home. Nine percent of all U.S. children have asthma, double the rate in the 1980s. Juvenile diabetes, obesity, and neurodevelopmental disorders have all increased alarmingly since then. According to a 2000 report in *Mental Health Information*, 18 percent of all American kids had a chronic condition, compared to 1.8 percent in 1960. That's a tenfold increase that is already translating into young adults with costlier health care needs than ever before. For the first time in our history, our children's life expectancy will be shorter than our own. Having a chronic health problem or a developmental disability often goes hand in hand with myriad nutrition issues, and these can make your child more vulnerable to infections and illness.

This is where nutrition plays a starring role. Nutrition status in children predicts whether infections and illnesses are acute or mild, frequent or rare, life-threatening or survivable. It literally prevents mortality from infections in children—by more than 50 percent according to some global data. We've all been ingrained to wholly credit vaccinations for this. But there are many illustrations of how much nutrition matters for the immune function of babies and kids, in our rich record of nutrition science. Weak nutrition status in an infant or young child heightens the risk of death from infections, regardless of vaccination status. This makes sense when we pause to remember basic nutrition science and the decades of data we have on public health nutrition from all over the globe. Even mild nutrition deficits contribute significantly to child mortality: Undernutrition is responsible for over five million deaths from infection that occur in low- and middle-income countries each year, in children under age five. What that means is, if these children had been in normal nutrition status, they would not have died from infections. Strong nutrition would help them fight back, or not get sick in the first place. Sadly, the United States is now a country with more hunger and food insecurity than you might think, with overlap between kids who have both a special need and food insecurity. More than seventeen million children in America receive food stamp benefits. For many, a lunch courtesy of the federally funded school lunch program is their only, or their most nutritious, meal of the day.

Whether those meals are nutritious at all is a discussion unto itself, as schools struggle to deliver healthy food to young learners with limited kitchen facilities, tight budgets, and commodity foods that are actually refused by the likes of Kentucky Fried Chicken and McDonald's.

It's also plain how much nutrition status matters when we remember that vaccines are meant to *provoke* an immune response—they don't *provide* the actual molecules, cells, structures, and protein components that the immune system needs to control infection. These components are fabricated with nutrients extracted from food, not from the contents of that vaccine syringe at the well-baby checkup. Whether the exposure is natural or from a vaccine, the immune system responds by drawing from its pool of available nutrients. Infants and children who have chronic inflammation, who are in meager status for total calories or total protein, who are underweight, or who lack individual nutrients such as iron, zinc, or vitamins A and D will remain more vulnerable to infection. Meanwhile, children with special needs who have difficulty getting all the nutrition they need from their diets are in the same boat: They may be underweight, overweight, lacking certain nutrients, or not absorbing nutrients very well. This can put them in the same nutritional risk category as kids who experience chronic malnutrition from lack of reliable access to good food intakes and hunger. And *that* means more frequent and more severe illnesses and infections.

Nutrition-focused tools are easy to use for minimizing infections and illness. Usually when children enter my practice and start working with these, they experience a winter with no illness, or much less illness than in the past. Parents are often surprised with this "side effect" of nutrition care. To my view, this isn't a surprise; it's normal. This is what strong nutrition status can and should do for your children. This doesn't mean your child will never get sick, but it does mean your child's immune system can function more as intended. Here's where to start:

Remove inflammatory foods. Think your child has no inflammation from foods? Think again—especially if your pediatrician or allergist was suspicious enough about this to do some testing but found nothing, or if your child experiences colds, viruses, flu, pneumonia, asthma, or ear infections each year. Correct assessment of inflammation from foods is a common oversight in pediatric practice today. It's probably the one that parents ask me about most often. While the medical community usually acknowledges that food allergies matter, concern and interest tend to stop there, once testing for food allergies is done. Your allergist most likely screened only for the most obvious of immune responses, with a test called RAST. This can be done with a skin prick or a blood test. In either case, the immune response looked for here is an antibody called Immunoglobulin E, or IgE. When IgE is problematic, kids may have hives, vomiting, stomachaches, skin rashes, loose stools from a trigger food, or tingling in the lips and mucosal lining of the mouth and throat. They can also have severe IgE responses that warrant carrying an EpiPen, or trips to the emergency room with accidental exposures to trigger foods. Tests can check for total IgE level (measuring all your body's IgE antibody to anything and everything) or IgE to individual triggers (measuring IgE only to triggers chosen, such as grasses, nuts, milk, pollen, strawberries, trees, etc.). If you found some positives on the panel, you can work from there to decide how to organize and prioritize your child's food intake. If nothing was found, and your child still gets sick often, is leaning toward ADD or ADHD signs, has autism or mood disorders, has stomachaches, shiners, irritability, picky appetite, or irritable mixed stools, then you may need to do more digging with an ELISA test for IgG—read on.

Our immune systems have more than one way to react to stuff, so just looking at the one most obvious response to foods by checking IgE is only part of the story. In fact, immune function is so complex and intelligent that how it works still isn't fully understood—especially when it comes to esoteric tools such as homeopathy and acupuncture. Benefits have been documented from these modalities, but Western medical science can't yet describe how or why they work. We do know that when the immune system misconstrues a benign food protein fragment as an invader to be destroyed, something is awry. This means the immune system is wasting its resources mounting a response to something that can't infect you or really invade your body. If that "something" is dairy protein—which is in milk, yogurt, cheese, ice cream, and so on—or anything else your child eats a lot of every day, then your child's immune system is very busy fighting nothing even when he *isn't* sick. It also means that when a true pathogen rolls in, such as this winter's flu bug, his immune system has weaker, less organized resources to fight back. Add to this a meager cache of resources in the first place because of nutrition deficits, and you have a child who probably gets sick a lot.

If you have never had food allergy testing but note that your child has some of the problems listed below on a chronic basis, start by requesting a RAST (IgE) screening with your primary provider for any suspect foods. If you don't suspect any particular food, start with the usual culprits, which are dairy protein, wheat protein (gluten), tree nuts, peanut, soy, eggs, and corn. Kids with these symptoms on a regular basis likely have inflammation that is not well controlled:

- Asthma events

- Frequent upper respiratory infections

- Upper respiratory infections that advance to pneumonia

- Frequent tiredness, malaise, or lethargy*

- Chronic congestion in the nose and throat

- Ear infections

- Chronic stooling problems (can't potty train, stool incontinence after potty training, mixed hard and loose stools, constipation, or chronic wet/irritable stools)

- Chronic stomachaches, headaches, vomiting, or reflux

- Unexplained eczema, hives, or rashes

If you find some foods with moderate to high reactivity on your child's RAST test, remove them from his diet. You will need to replace these foods with new ones of equal or better nutritional value. If you only find one, lucky you! Remove it. If you find two, remove them. If you find more than two, start prioritizing. You can't remove more than three or four foods from a child's diet

---

* These can also signal anemia, low iron status, low total calories, or other nutrition problems.

without using special medical foods or supplement supports to restore the high-value protein and calorie sources you are losing. I have encountered many parents in a tizzy because they were told to remove *all* foods showing *any* reactivity from an allergy panel. Don't do it—it doesn't work to do this in children, because children are growing. The injury you will inflict by using an overly restrictive diet is too great; without professional intervention, your child's food intake will not be adequate to support new tissue growth and repair along with all the other demands on a child's growing body and developing brain. Children who truly must remove four, five, eight, or *all* intact proteins from their diets need professional supervision. Get a referral from your pediatrician for a nutrition assessment. In these cases, amino acid–based formulas and protein sources are a necessity, not an option, as are thoughtful strategies to provide adequate calories from carbohydrates and fats, which spare the protein for priority jobs such as tissue growth and repair, neurotransmitter construction, immune function, and much more. Products that use low-inflammatory proteins such as rice protein powder can be used in some cases, as long as the rice protein source is augmented properly with essential amino acids (rice is a low-quality protein that needs boosting in order to be of value to humans). When managing several inflammatory foods, your strategy to reduce inflammation must expand to rely on more than just removing trigger foods.

Besides removing the two or three most inflammatory foods, rotate foods that are less triggering. Add supplements that help control inflammation, such as probiotics, liposomal glutathione, and omega-3 fats. Protein that is in a free amino acid form has also been shown to help gut tissue repair in children with Crohn's disease; add this to your child's morning smoothie, hot cereal, or favorite soft food. See page 249 for a meal replacement recipe that includes free essential amino acids.

Frequency of exposure matters here, too; your goal is lowering the total inflammatory load on the immune system. So if your child is highly reactive (but not anaphylactic with hives) to lemons and strawberries, but moderately reactive to gluten or wheat, it's more important to remove the wheat. Why? Because your child probably eats wheat many times a day and relies on it as a major protein and calorie source, while those fruits are probably eaten a lot less frequently. The wheat may trigger lower-intensity inflammation, but it is being triggered a lot more often, leading to chronic inflammation, which you need to stop.

What if your child rejects the new foods he needs to eat, and pines with a fury for his old favorites? It's never easy to take away favorite foods, so don't expect your child to be agreeable. See *Special-Needs Kids Eat Right* for more information on strategies for shifting appetites. Here's the very first one to consider: If your child is so picky that she adamantly won't accept new foods, then you likely have another problem—bowel infections. These reliably jam up appetites in children in my experience, and no amount of sneaky recipe tactics or behavior therapy budges this very far. Mixing nutritious ingredients into recipes is a great way to go, until you are mad at everybody in your house because you spent all day shopping, cooking, and messing up your kitchen only to have nobody eat your masterpiece. Of course, if it's working, stick with it—it's all about balancing what works for your family. Meanwhile, treating bowel infections, followed by checking that the treatment was successful, will help expand your child's appetite, improve absorption, and permit more nutritious foods to be included. See the discussion on bowel infections and appetite in Chapter 4.

Next, keep digging. Let's say your doctor did a RAST test, and it was negative—but your child still has active signs for inflammation from foods. Now what? The next layer of the immune response to foods should be checked. This is not a test that pediatricians and pediatric allergists "believe in," if I can quote what parents often tell me. I'm not sure where the "believe" part comes in; rather than take it on faith, I take it on the data, which shows that IgG-mediated food sensitivities can impair growth in infants and young children, and can trigger reflux and other GI symptoms. I have also observed that these responses can trigger sensory and mood irritability; interfere with attention, learning, and focus; and create a dull background roar of GI, skin, or respiratory symptoms. IgG is another immunoglobulin made by the immune system. Unlike IgE, it tends to have a slower onset with a less dramatic cluster of symptoms. The test that checks IgG is called ELISA, or enzyme linked immunosorbent assay. It is a blood test. Work with specialty labs that can check IgG reactions to several foods with little blood. Some labs use a finger stick test that requires only five blood spots; others can do over ninety foods with one 2-milliliter tube of blood. Your child should not have to give pints of blood to be screened for IgG reactions to foods.

So far, I have not encountered a major children's hospital gastroenterology unit anywhere in the United States that offers ELISA panels. Plenty of data now links IgG reactivity to gluten (wheat) with many skin, neurological, and GI symptoms. Other data shows that IgG responses to other foods may impair growth, lessen food intake, and cause other GI problems in infants and children. Parents always hope this test will be done by their gastroenterologist or pediatrician, and ask me to explain the test to their doctors. I demur. Other than a single screening for gluten sensitivity, I have not yet seen gastro docs or peds use ELISA in my ten-plus years in practice with children from states nationwide. The standard seems to be to offer IgE testing only, usually followed either by "I've never heard of that" when parents ask for IgG testing or a lecture for Mom and Dad on why other immune responses to foods don't matter. This is when I get to respectfully disagree with my clients' physicians and invite the opportunity to illustrate why, either with case histories or with assessing your own child's test results. I have noted that the Massachusetts General Pediatric Gastroenterology and Nutrition Unit may offer ELISA IgG to foods as individual tests, meaning lots more money and blood out of you and your child than is necessary, compared to using functional medicine labs that specialize in this by offering analysis of dozens of foods with a very small sample of blood. See the resources section for the names of labs that do this test.

Let's say you've found a few foods you need to pull from your child's diet, but you are unsure where to start. For an ingenious tool that lets you customize your child's special diet needs instantly into recipes, shopping lists, and menus, visit MyFoodMy Health.com and use the code SNKGPF (the initials of this book title) for a discount on your subscription, if you sign up. If you don't want to sign up for that service, mine this site for its wealth of free information and recipes from a team of professionals experienced with food allergies, functional medicine, cooking, and special diets. My Food My Health also supports my goal in practice to have the person in charge of cooking prepare meals *everyone* can eat—definitely easier and cheaper than crafting separate meals for separate kids, adults, appetites, and sensitivities. Families who do this don't have as much success with special diet strategies, in my experience. Other favorite web resources of mine for special diet planning are Renegade Kitchen (renegadekitchen.com), Will's Kitchen (willskitchen.com), and the Wheat-Free Gourmet (wheatfreegourmet.com). Renegade Kitchen's theme is good food for the "allergy bound." You will find a no-excuses, high-positivity take on good food, demonstrated with pictures and an engaging video, for all sorts of recipes that skip gluten, nuts, dairy, and other stuff. Will's Kitchen is a recipe blog, again with good visuals, that shuns eggs, dairy, and nuts. Wheat-Free Gourmet features a chef with Italian heritage and celiac disease, guiding readers through even the most complicated authentic Italian recipes. The Internet has many resources such as these to help your family eat well during cold and flu season. This is essential to good health and infection fighting. Be sure to see the resources section for notable cookbooks for special-needs eating, too. As you choose your favorite recipes from the infinite sources on the web and in books, follow these basic guidelines to keep your meals as nutritious and health promoting as possible:

When possible, go organic. Pesticides have degenerative neuro-toxic effects and are implicated as possibly contributing to Parkinson's disease. Acute exposures are clearly dangerous, but we are just beginning to realize that repetitive, low-dose exposures are likely contributing to chronic disease. Some researchers wonder if they are implicated in conditions such as ADHD, autism, or childhood cancers and chronic inflammatory conditions, too. Children, being small, are especially vulnerable; their exposures to environmental toxins are at an all-time high from foods, air, vaccines, plastics, and other sources. Research by the Environmental Working Group found that we may be able to lower exposure to agricultural toxins and pesticides by 80 percent, simply by choosing to buy these items from reputable organic growers: The most pesticide-laden foods are apples, cherries, grapes (imported from Chili), nectarines, peaches, pears, raspberries, strawberries, bell peppers, celery, potatoes, and spinach. Even after washing, studies showed that these produce items still contained significant pesticide residues. Consider this when you buy juices for your child as well.

Organic produce can have better nutrient profiles than conventional produce, especially for certain minerals and for vitamin C, depending on the water content of the food in question. Organic grains can vary, too: They may have less total protein in some cases, but the protein is of better value and is more nutritious (the levels of individual amino acids are higher). While you may have heard there is no difference between organic and conventionally raised crops, I disagree. This happened to be the subject of one of my graduate projects at the University of Hawaii in the 1980s, well before organics came back into vogue. At the time, organic food was an obscure and laughable throwback to the prior decade! Now that most major supermarkets prominently feature organic foods and entire chains have evolved around them, it's plain that organically raised crops are here to stay.

Buy organic milk, meat, chicken, and eggs if you can afford them. The nonorganic versions of these foods don't have as much pesticide residue as produce items do, but they have a greater *variety* of agricultural chemicals. They can contain antibiotic and hormone residues along with fertilizer and pesticide residues used on feed grains. Fatty acid profiles of eggs and meats that are raised organically are healthier. Beef cattle are normally fed pesticide-laden corn when raised conventionally. Grass is their native food; grass-fed beef has less total fat per serving and more omega-3 fats. The same can be true for chickens and eggs: When raised on pasture, their meat and eggs contain many times more healthy omega-3 fats than when they are raised in indoor factories. Omega-3 fats support anti-inflammatory prostaglandin production in the body, while trans fats, too many polyunsaturated fats, or hydrogenated and saturated fats can tilt prostaglandins toward inflammation. Wild-caught fish are also higher in healthy oils than farm-raised fish, which may be fed grains such as corn. The best marine sources of omega-3s are wild salmon, halibut, scallops, and shrimp, as well as krill and algae. You can choose foods like these that supply omega-3s, in addition to taking an omega-3 supplement. If you are avoiding fish, try algae sources, flax oil (organic preferably), ground flaxseed, walnuts if tolerated, edamame (boiled soybeans), tofu, or winter squash.

Get a slow cooker or Dutch oven. Use high-quality organic ingredients to slowly simmer or roast meats, poultry, and vegetables with any combo of seasonings. It's easy to set this up in the morning and let it cook all day for a nutrient-rich meal. Minerals, proteins, and healthy fats will abound in a slow-cooked soup, stew, or roast. By dinnertime all you will need is to add some bread on the side, even if it's gluten-free. If you have enough broth, stir penne pasta in for the last half hour for your own variation on minestrone. Another easy-assembly meal is rolled pork roast covered with sliced onion, bell pepper, and sweet potato, with a smothering of a favorite barbecue sauce, baked covered until done (usually about fifty minutes, depending on the size of the roast). This is accompanied nicely by quinoa or rice.

Keep favorite broths on hand. You can buy ready-to-use, organic broths made from beef, chicken, or vegetables. They don't require refrigeration until opened. These help make fast meals if you didn't get to set up a stew or soup earlier. Sauté your vegetables until soft first, in olive oil with garlic or favorite seasonings; add meat or tofu; then add broth and let simmer for fifteen minutes. Save bones or hocks from hams, chicken, or other butcher items you buy to make your own broths, if you can.

Use lots of fresh ginger root, garlic, and onion. Ginger has strong antioxidant and anti-inflammatory capabilities, which some say rival nonsteroidal anti-inflammatory drugs such as ibuprofen. It is a mainstay of Chinese medicine. Steep a few slices in hot chicken broth along with minced scallion, cilantro, fresh ground pepper, and soft tofu chunks to sip when congested with cold or flu, or add a slice to hot tea. Try it in a miso (fermented soy) broth, if your child can tolerate soy. If your child likes hot chocolate but has a dairy allergy or trouble with a phenolic food such as chocolate, he might love a spicy chai with acai syrup instead of sugar, ginger root, and steamed milk that is on the safe list, such as hemp, almond, or coconut milk. Garlic and onion both have antimicrobial effects that can be quite potent when you use them fresh (rather than powdered versions, pills, or supplements—unless you are purchasing a specific extract tested for potency). Just typing "garlic" into the National Library of Medicine database yields more than 3,200 research articles discussing its antimicrobial action, antioxidant properties, benefits in heart disease, and more—including the ability of garlic extract to slow formation of fibrotic tissue in the liver! Onions or their extracts have been shown to decrease bronchial spasms in asthma, to provide healthy fructo-oligosaccharide prebiotics for beneficial bowel flora, to slow tumor growth, and to deliver antimicrobial agents strong enough to kill organisms that may cause food-borne illnesses such as *E. coli*, bacillus, and salmonella. Imagine a rich onion soup made with organic beef broth—a definitely soothing, and perhaps even healing, meal for cold and flu season. Or try fresh finely minced garlic tumbled on Udi's gluten-free pizza rounds (my favorite), smeared with lots of olive oil and a good dash of salt. These bake fast (ten or twelve minutes) and are a delicious cold weather treat alone or as a side to soups and stews.

Maximize sensible supplements. If you haven't heard about vitamin D's role in preventing flu, cancers, upper respiratory infections, and many other conditions, it's time to get caught up on the latest research findings. Vitamin D was overlooked for decades as nothing other than the vitamin that prevents rickets, and since nearly nobody had rickets (until recently), nobody paid much attention. Then, around the turn of this century, pediatricians began noticing rickets again in infants and young children, putting the spotlight back on vitamin D. Data showed that much of the population of North America was vitamin D deficient (based on blood work done on 19,000 adults nationwide). It was also found that, compared to earlier data, vitamin D levels had slid downward over the last twenty or thirty years; in the same time frame, many chronic diseases got worse, including skin cancer. Paradoxically, the culprit may have been years of avoiding sunlight, using more sunscreen, and staying indoors; exposure to sun permits us to generate the bioactive form of vitamin D through a reaction in skin. Breast-fed babies were found to be more vulnerable, since they didn't take vitamin D–fortified formula, and since moms were likely deficient in this nutrient, too.

In response to all this, the Institute of Medicine's Food and Nutrition Board revisited its recommendations for daily intake of vitamin D, and decided they were far too low—only enough to permit normal bone formation, but not enough to help prevent a host of other conditions and diseases, from impaired immune response to heart disease. A short list of conditions correlating with low vitamin D status includes increased risk for falls in elderly people, increased risk for several types of cancer including skin cancer, diabetes, and more upper respiratory infections or flu. While vaccination against flu has not shown terribly stellar performance for prevention, vitamin D has: Poor vitamin D status will considerably magnify your child's vulnerability to lung infections, especially for kids with chronic lung conditions such as asthma or cystic fibrosis.

A flurry of research activity has sprung up around vitamin D in the last decade. More a signaling hormone than a vitamin, it has been found to play a key role in immune signaling and even gene expression. Government guidelines for daily intakes have been upped considerably for kids—from a couple hundred international units (IU) to 1000 or 2000 per day. Many physicians and researchers advocate using even more. Infants who are breast-fed should be given 1000 international units of vitamin D daily, and you can easily obtain supplements at any pharmacy, supermarket, or vitamin shop. Use concentrated drops of vitamin D3; these usually deliver 1000 international units per drop. Children above age one year should be given at least 2000 international units daily. In winter, consider increasing their dose to 5000 international units per day. Your pediatrician can order a blood test for your child if you want to be sure about the dosage needed. Vitamin D has very low toxicity and it is difficult to overdo it, especially if you live in a cold climate and spend most of your winter inside or under coats and hats. Have your own level checked if you are breast-feeding, and let your doctor correct it with a supplement recommendation; research suggests you will need at least 6000 international units per day to raise levels in your breast milk. In some cases, physicians will give much larger doses on a weekly basis to correct very low levels.

Vitamin D may turn out to be the single most important nutrient you could supplement, especially in winter months. It isn't easy to get from food, and the sun is too low in much of North America in winter for us to benefit from it. You can add cod liver oil, lots of fish, or fortified foods such as milk—but these are foods some of us are avoiding because of allergies or concerns about mercury. Cod liver oil can be purchased from reputable companies, such as Nordic Naturals, that screen carefully for toxins and heavy metals. Supplemental drops are easy to use.

What other nutrients are notable for children with special health and developmental concerns, when it comes to staying infection-free? Minerals such as iron and zinc have a clear impact on susceptibility to infections and the vigor of immune responses. Minerals are easy to deplete if your child has been eating a "white" diet for a while—that is, mac and cheese, pizza, milk, yogurt confections, refined breads, bagels, pastas, ice cream, and sweets. These foods come up empty for supplying most any minerals (except calcium from the dairy foods). They are short on magnesium, selenium, chromium, zinc, iodine, and iron. Even if you give your child a chewable multivitamin, read the label and you will find that most of these deliver vitamins, but only a small percentage of some (not all) recommended minerals. Minerals also regulate countless chemical reactions in cells that manage everything from nerve impulse transmission to blood sugar levels.

If your child avoids mineral-rich foods such as organic pork, beef, vegetables, dark greens, nuts, dates, or fermented soy foods such as tempeh or miso, you can at least give him a complete supplement that includes some of the daily recommended intake for each mineral (no multi can provide a complete dose of all the minerals needed—the pills would be enormous, and individuals vary widely for doses of minerals needed or tolerated). Pediatricians can screen for poor status for iron and other minerals with blood tests if necessary, but signs in children are fairly obvious when minerals are lacking. They include:

- A food intake that generally excludes mineral-rich foods

- Kids over age one year who drink more than 25–30 ounces of milk per day

- Pallor, dark circles under the eyes, or skin that looks translucent (see veins through skin)

- Chewing or eating ice, dirt, or sand

- Mouthing or chewing nonfood items routinely

- Teeth grinding

- White dots on fingernails, ridges in nails

- Thyroid imbalances

- Wider than normal blood sugar swings (per readings on an instrument such as AccuChek)

- Hyperactivity, mood irritability, impulsivity, insomnia

- Cracked skin or cuts that heal too slowly

Of all the minerals, iron is perhaps the most intriguing. We have ingenious mechanisms in the body to balance how much of this critical nutrient we absorb from foods, how much we store, and how much we excrete. It is needed by all living cells, including bacteria and microbes, but it is also toxic or lethal if overdosed. For children with chronic inflammatory conditions, Crohn's or celiac disease, or bowel infections—such as some now noted in children with autism—iron absorption will be impaired. Besides impairing immune response, iron deficiency anemia causes motor delays, attention and behavior problems, and even diminishes social interaction. A healthy intestine signals the body on when to absorb more iron from food and when not to. Most children in my practice—and many special-needs children in general—show some type of problem absorbing diets normally, and/or bowel infections such as *Helicobacter pylori*, candida and other fungal species such as rhodotorula, or flourishing klebsiella and clostridia species when I test them with stool cultures. They also may not have healthy tissue in the duodenum, the part of the intestine responsible for this iron-balancing act, owing to years of inflammation from foods or nasty microbes. Several kids in my practice have already been "scoped"—that is, they've undergone endoscopy, a procedure in which a gastroenterologist peers into the digestive tract with a tiny camera. Many do show tissue changes in the duodenum, and in other places along their GI tracts. It's surprising that these kids are not typically referred for a nutrition assessment or a screening for mineral status, an essential to good health. Tell your provider team that you want these nutrition points screened for your child, if you are seeing problems listed in this chapter.

Chronic inflammation can reduce iron uptake, creating anemia. Babies who have cow's milk sensitivity, as well as older kids with inflammatory bowel disease, will lose iron to microscopic, chronic bleeding in the GI tract. Bowel infections that cause the gut wall integrity to suffer or that injure our mechanism to control iron uptake may permit *too much* iron into circulation. Giving supplemental iron when bowel infections are florid, or when blood sugar is poorly controlled, can cause havoc, too: The iron feeds bacteria and microbes handily. Some research (and loads of anecdotal reports) shows that these bowel infections drive behaviors and features of autism, mood swings, and ADHD. I have witnessed iron supplements trigger violent, aggressive behavior in at least two boys with autism, who had untreated bowel infections.

To sum up, if your child has signs of weakened iron status or actual iron deficiency anemia, clear out the bowel infections before using iron supplements. Have your doctor check ferritin, total iron binding capacity (TIBC), red blood cell count, shape, and size (a "CBC" panel), and hemoglobin to define your child's overall iron status, so the dosing can be safely chosen. Other special-needs circumstances deserving mention here are children with Type 1 diabetes, or children with autism spectrum disorders. Too much iron can damage the pancreas, and its output of insulin, if the body has trouble controlling how much iron it absorbs. So it is wise for kids with diabetes to only use iron supplements with monitoring by their endocrinologist. For kids with autism, the same question of iron toxicity has been raised, but barely studied. I have met many children on the spectrum who needed and benefited from iron supplements, but there are others who may not handle iron uptake normally. Iron toxicity to brain and nerve tissue is a possibility in these children; once again, have your provider thoroughly assess iron status—this means checking both iron stores and circulating, available iron for your child. Children with chronic inflammatory conditions can develop anemia by virtue of how body chemistry changes in the context of inflammation, so those with asthma, cystic fibrosis, frequent infections, or multiple food allergies will need thoughtful assessment of iron status also, before adding an iron supplement.

The next important nutrition tool to keep immune function strong is the right protein intake, healthfully absorbed—and for children, this must be taken in the context of adequate total calories. Protein eaten without enough energy from other sources (fat or carbohydrate) is essentially destroyed so it can be used to meet energy needs, which are higher in children because: They are growing! Remember? They are not little adults, so diets that skimp too much on healthy carbs, whose calories mostly come from raw or fermented foods, or that source most calories from protein are more likely to impair growth, cognition, and some of your child's body chemistry. Using protein for energy is a metabolically inefficient process that renders it useless for other tasks that only protein can achieve, such as tissue construction, immune molecule production, or manufacture of all kinds of signaling chemicals, hormones, neurotransmitters, or cell structures. Children who eat most of their calories from protein tend to have growth impairments, lesser bone density, and may end up with increased risk for certain cancers—so too much of it is not a good thing.

On the other hand, too little of it is common in diets of kids with food allergies, reflux, or weak, picky appetites. They may not eat enough protein, and may have trouble digesting it. Under normal circumstances, children need anywhere from 1 gram to 1.5 grams of protein per kilogram of body weight per day; a little less is fine; a little more is fine, too. By way of example, if your child only eats 20 grams of protein daily, this is not fine (unless we are talking about a very small person, such as a young infant). If your child eats in excess of 100 grams of protein on a daily basis, this is also not fine. While true protein deficiency is rare in the United States, children with special health care needs or food insecurity are at risk for poor protein intakes, and this makes them more vulnerable to infections. The amount of protein that is best for a child varies by age, weight, status for other nutrition concerns, or growth pattern, so it's difficult to give blanket recommendations. But look for these signs, which suggest a possible deficit for protein:

- Slowing progress on the height-for-age curve on the growth chart

- Thinning hair

- Hair that lacks luster and appears dull, or falls out easily

- Hair that seems to grow very slowly or very little

- Soft, peeling, or easily cracked nails

- Anemia

- Changes in thyroid chemistry

- Fatigue

- Pale skin that appears thin

- A wasted appearance with a bloated belly

- Slower than expected onset of puberty

- Lethargy with muscle weakness

If after checking these signs, you're still not sure whether your child is eating enough protein, get a referral from your doctor for a nutrition assessment. A dietitian can calculate for you whether or not your child's food intake meets his needs. You can also use supplements for protein, if it is hard for your child to eat enough. If allergies or sensitivities are an issue, do allergy (IgE) and sensitivity (IgG) testing first, so you know which foods are safe and non-inflammatory. If lab testing is not an option with your doctor, check a site called Direct Labs on the web and talk to an MD support person there about getting the testing done.

Using Protein Supplements

It surprises me how often children are told to add a protein supplement by well-meaning providers, when the inflammatory loads from foods have not been assessed first. Protein powders are often problematic for children with food allergies or sensitivities, which is why some testing first can be helpful. Whether you've had the benefit of allergy or sensitivity testing first or not, if you would like to introduce a protein supplement, use a small dose to start, at a time when your child is home with no demands or scheduled activities, so you can watch for a reaction (stomachache; irritability; hives; tingling of the lips, tongue, or throat; or vomiting and diarrhea). Protein supplements can be mixed into soft foods and smoothies, and are usually made from egg, whey, whole milk protein, soy, and rice. Rice protein powders have poor nutritional value, and should be augmented with at least one amino acid—lysine—in order to provide adequate nutritional support. For the same reason, children can't rely on milks from rice, hemp, almond, or coconut for protein. What little protein they do contain is of poor quality, lacking some of the amino acids that are essential to humans. Use these in baking, cooking, or as a smoothie base, and augment them with supplemental protein powders that you know your child can tolerate. Consider specialized elemental formulas such as Neocate or Elecare (available powdered or ready to drink) if you've tried dairy-based formulas such as Ensure or Boost without success. These are discussed in more detail in the resources section.

Add Zinc

Round out your immune booster nutrients with enough zinc. Your child's multivitamin probably delivers 5–10 milligrams of zinc, which is fine as long as she eats a great diet that includes zinc-rich foods (many kids don't). Add a zinc lozenge, liquid zinc, or a separate chewable, or foods such as shellfish, wheat germ, sesame tahini, organically raised beef and pork, chickpeas or hummus, or pumpkin seeds. Clinical signs peculiar to poor zinc status are teeth grinding (in sleep or awake), mouthing nonfood objects, biting (as in biting other people or peers), streaks or dots on nails, slow healing of wounds or cuts, delay in onset of puberty, weak appetite—even acne can improve if low zinc is replenished. Children can use supplements starting at 20 milligrams daily; special

circumstances may merit using more. Since zinc and iron compete for absorption, don't dose these two supplements together if
you can help it. Using higher doses of zinc (30 milligrams per day
and up) for the long term can drive down the iron status in a child.
If your child needs additional zinc, such as is used in chelation
therapy protocols or in many autism supplement protocols, have
your provider periodically check iron status and adjust your supplement regimen accordingly.

The Importance of Vitamin A

The final nutrient to highlight here, when it comes to infection
fighting and immune function, is vitamin A. Vitamin A is effective
as a preventive and treatment for measles and other viral infections; it has a lengthy pedigree in the scientific literature for this,
so much so that the World Health Organization has a protocol that
describes dosages to use in children who are depleted. Depletion
of this nutrient makes children more susceptible to viral infections.
In the United States, where milk and other foods are fortified with
this nutrient, vitamin A deficiency is not very common—but intakes of this nutrient are too low for nearly half the population,
according to surveillance data. Vitamin A foods include anything
fortified with it (milk, juices), or deeply colored fruits and vegetables. If those foods are problematic for your child because of allergies or because of phenols, add ½ teaspoon of cod liver oil to the
daily regimen. This gives a modest daily dose of vitamin A along
with omega-3 fatty acids and a spot of vitamin D (about 60 international units or less). Buy a reputable brand that is tightly quality controlled for mercury and other contaminants, and look for

natural antioxidants in it such as vitamin E, to help the flavor stay tolerable. Many cod liver oil products are available now for kids, with flavors such as citrus, strawberry, or peach, to make it easy to take daily. Vitamin A is another nutrient (like iron, some other minerals, or vitamins E, D, and K) that the body can store, making it toxic if taken to excess. How much a child needs depends on his weight, current vitamin A status, and whether or not he is managing a virus. Don't supplement your child with more than 5000 international units of vitamin A daily for more than a month without professional guidance. If you've been supplementing this vitamin or using cod liver oil for a while, you might suspect vitamin A toxicity in a child whose appetite has diminished, or who complains of pain in the long bones or shins, has suddenly thinning hair for no other likely reason, has night sweats, or who has a dry crackle-glaze look on his skin.

Probiotics, again. For warding off stomach flu bugs, a maintenance regimen that includes a probiotic supplement may help. Probiotics can be taken in this way long term, for months at a time. Others are best for shorter duration. For example, if your child gets a stomach flu, consider a supplemental microbe called *Saccharomyces boulardii*, as soon as her tender stomach allows. *S. boulardii*—known as "Sac B" for short—has shown clinical success literally the world over for fighting intestinal infections. Research focuses on its strength in ridding our intestines of unwanted bacterial pathogens as well as some viral strains such as rotavirus. Sac B generally does not like to populate a human gut, and will work to eradicate unwanted species, then leave as well. But continual supplementation may permit it to situate in the gut and cause fungal overgrowth of its own, which is not desirable. White patchy material in your child's stool may signal this, so it is probably advisable to withdraw Sac B if you note this—and as always, let your provider know. Additional signs of fungal infection are itchy red groin area or diaper rash, bed-wetting in a potty-trained child, or mood irritability and reactivity. Sac B is available at most better supplement shops. It is reasonable to use this for up to a month at the most, but not as a long-term maintenance microbe. Switch back to the lactobacillus or bifidobacteria species for that job. If your child struggles on these, talk to a professional for guidance. Some children in my practice—especially those who relied on antacids and reflux medications in infancy and toddlerhood—seem to have more trouble populating their intestines with microflora that is normally helpful to us, and may need another strategy or product.

Annual flu shots. Many special-needs kids have circumstances that place them on the priority list for getting flu shots when the new ones come out, year after year. Is this the best defense to offer your child? You might be surprised to hear about a comprehensive Cochrane review done in 2009 that looked at hundreds of studies on what works best to prevent flu: shots or physical barriers? "Physical barriers" included hand washing, quarantine (that is, just staying home), and various types of face masks. The review found that flu vaccines worked no better than physical barriers to prevent the spread of influenza. Though this review did not assess the literature for impact of nutrition tools, such as vitamin D, on influenza, other research has. By most any accounts, this is one nutrient whose performance is turning out to be nothing short of spectacular, owing to its very low toxicity and its broad sweep on many facets of body chemistry. Flu infections have always reliably happened more in winter months; new research is attributing this to sun exposure, which we get much less of in winter, thus depleting the body's vitamin D stockpile. Special-needs children who are less able to run around outdoors daily at any time of year, regardless of weather and sunlight, are at even higher risk. Supplementing vitamin D handily prevents this depletion.

Another surprise about flu vaccines is that since their introduction in the 1970s, deaths caused by flu have increased, not decreased, and the variety and virulence of influenza is increasing, not diminishing. The total number of influenza-like illnesses reported by providers to the CDC more than quadrupled between 1997 and 2006, according to the CDC's own data. So if flu vaccines are truly the miraculous elixirs we hope they are, why is flu increasing? It's certain that our population is aging, with more elderly citizens around than ever, and these individuals *are* susceptible when it comes to flu, but this doesn't fully explain the increase in flu deaths or virulence. Flu shots still contain mercury, aluminum, or other unwanted adjuvants and preservatives, which lead some to favor the proven natural immune supports such as vitamin D, normal mineral status (especially for iron and zinc), and adequate diets that avoid inflammatory foods. After a decade in practice, I've witnessed that nutrition-focused tools described here are reliable and safe preventives for flu, compared to annual vaccination. We also have a venerable and well-pedigreed data set that shows how crucial good nutrition status is for infants and children, when it comes to preventing infection. Do your own research and reading, to satisfy yourself on what is best for your family. Input from your providers—both those who rely on vaccines in practice and those who apply other tools—can help guide you.

The Pharm-Free Tools Are Many

Findings can be cited to highlight each and every individual vitamin and mineral, in terms of how they support immune function. The ones covered in this chapter have, based on my own observation in practice, the biggest impact for children managing special needs. Nutrition tools are only as good as their weakest piece; like an intricate web, they all depend on each other to deliver the best for our health. Focusing on one tool at the expense of the others doesn't work well; for example, children who use many supplements but who have poor food intakes will not derive hoped-for benefits from all those pills. And children using lots of supplements may not be benefiting at all, which is why some professional guidance is a good idea. Maximize and organize nutrition tools to keep your kids healthy, no matter what special challenges they may have, and get professional input. Check my own site, NutritionCare.net, if you have questions or need support. Engage a naturopathic doctor (ND) who is practiced in working with babies and kids to bring in the pharmacopeia of safe, infection-fighting, or immune-boosting herbal tools such as olive leaf extract, calendula, astragalus, or echinacea, to name just a few. Like medications, these natural tools are best approached with professional supervision. For example, children with inflammatory conditions should use goldenseal or echinacea carefully, as they up-regulate immune response. Check with a classical homeopath on remedies that might treat stomach flu with violent diarrhea or vomiting (try Arsenicum); stomach bugs that still hurt even after vomiting (treat with Ipecachua); congestion and colds (use Allium); or sudden hot fevers and fast-rising viral infections that quickly flush your child's cheeks (give

Belladonna). There are hundreds of remedies for professional homeopaths to choose from, which show efficacy in shortening the course and lessening severity of illnesses in many cases. Use these with professional guidance, and you will find that they can be quite effective—in some cases better—than pharmaceutical tools that have unwanted side effects.

Chapter Four

Growth Impairments, Underweight, and Overweight

GROWING STRONG WITH THE HEALTHIEST PATTERN FOR *YOUR* CHILD

"He's just little, that's what they said." Or: "It's because of his developmental diagnosis; it's just how he grows." How often I have heard that! But is it true? And even if it is, is it right for your child to remain "just little," or to "just grow this way"? Nutrition assessment tools that have been around for decades can help you find out, and can help you discern what to do. Being "little," underweight, or overweight are common problems for kids with special needs, who face hurdles for absorbing diets normally, eating normally, eliminating normally, or getting adequate exercise.

Growth patterns in children are easy to troubleshoot. That is what growth charts are for. Though someone at your child's pediatrician or specialist's office may dutifully put those dots on the chart at each visit, have you ever noticed they usually don't do anything with that information? I have met children entrenched in growth failure who come to my office after months—even years—of close monitoring with GI specialists who did nothing to troubleshoot why the child wasn't growing well. Common interventions are referrals to endocrinology for growth hormone injections (which may do little, or may not be needed at all, if the problem isn't growth hormone), or telling the family to use lots of fatty dairy foods or casein-based formulas to add calories. Neither of these look at *why* the child can't eat enough to grow, or can't grow well even when he's eating enough. Even when these tools fail, often nothing else is offered, other than the inevitable feeding tube, which will simply force more of the same poorly absorbed calories into the child.

Growth charts are great tools, and (in my opinion) they are underutilized in pediatrics today. Those dots, when regarded as a trend rather than individual dots, can say a lot about whether your child may need allergy testing, stool microbiology testing, more total calories, or more total protein—even what type of protein. They lend clues to when the trouble started and why. Was it around the time of vaccinations? Which one? Was it after a few rounds of antibiotics? Was it when solids, such as gluten, were introduced? Or was it even sooner, when infant formula was used? Working with this information helps me build an effective nutrition care plan that in most cases will turn a child's growth pattern around, prevent the feeding tube, or give a good boost to overall functional ability. For kids who need to lower their body mass index (BMI)—that is, they weigh too much, relative to their height—the growth chart can be just as useful for discerning when the overweight trend began, why, and how to remedy it. Getting children to lose weight should not be attempted without help from a dietitian or pediatrician—kids are still growing, and you need to carefully provide for all their nutrition needs, while addressing overweight.

Why scrutinize growth patterns? After all, we didn't used to pay so much attention to whether kids were too skinny or too fat. It matters now, though, because many *more* children are overweight than in the 1960s to 1980s, and this means higher rates of other chronic health problems associated with obesity that tend to become lifelong if left uncorrected before adulthood. There are also more medically fragile, underweight, and failure-to-thrive children than there used to be, secondary to myriad feeding and allergy problems that are skyrocketing today. Once growth problems are identified correctly, the right steps can be taken to restore what's healthy for a child. This isn't expensive to do or complicated. Correctly assessing and naming growth impairments can help trigger insurance coverage for nutrition care, but many parents—and even pediatricians—may not realize this. I recently called in to a radio talk show here in Colorado, when controversy popped up about a toddler denied health insurance because of her low weight. The ethics of the insurance provider were in question. They simply refused to cover the child at all. I explained that it is cost-effective to repair this with professional nutrition care. Denying care meant the child's risk for infections, for learning and developmental problems, and even for death would rise, ultimately costing more in the long run than preventive care.

Families can leverage these realities of nutrition status for children, to lower health care costs. Because this child was under age three, this insurance denial—made solely on the basis of her being underweight—may have qualified her for government health benefits under Medicaid. The federal government's Early Intervention Program, which includes a nutrition mandate, covers children ages zero to three, regardless of income status. Parents are entitled to access care with a registered dietitian under this program (I provide services in Colorado under this program). If you think your child may need nutrition care but you aren't sure where to turn, ask your pediatrician for an in-network referral, or contact your local Early Intervention Program yourself. This federal program operates with state matching funds under local program names from state to state—but each state has Early Intervention Funds, and a nutrition mandate is part of that funding. This is different from WIC (Women, Infants, and Children Supplemental Food Program), which qualifies children and families based on income, and provides nutrition education and food coupons. Early Intervention qualifies children based on a developmental concern, not income, and provides home-based services.

Early Intervention has been funded for decades because it works. We know how critical it is for infants and toddlers to be well nourished in the first three years of life, and how important it is for any developmental concerns to be redirected as early as possible with appropriate education, speech, or other therapies. These tools enhance life outcomes for children. If you would like to learn more about resources in your area for children ages zero to three, visit the website for the National Dissemination Center for Children with Disabilities (NICHCY.org) and click on "Help Babies (0–3)."

Roadblocks to Your Child's Healthy Growth Pattern: What They Mean

Underweight. Children are clinically underweight when they have a body mass index (BMI) below the 10th percentile for age, and they have "failure to thrive" (FTT) when they are below the 5th percentile for age for BMI. You can check your child's BMI right now by using the CDC's BMI calculator for teens and kids on the CDC website (cdc.gov/healthyweight/assessing/bmi). Or simply Google the phrase "BMI CDC" and follow links to this easy resource. If your child's BMI is hovering around the 10th percentile or lower, it's probably time to do something about it. Premies or kids who were born at around 6 pounds may be expected to progress along the bottom of the chart. But if your child was born above the 30th percentile for weight (about 7 pounds or higher), he ought to follow that trend through infancy, give or take a few points. If this is not happening, intervene; there is no need to wait until things worsen dramatically, when they are harder to reverse, because babies are vulnerable to developmental and morbidity impacts when they fall into growth regression or failure to thrive.

Failure to thrive. Both babies and older children may have FTT. As mentioned above, this means they've dropped to the bottom of the chart, or disappeared off the chart entirely. In my experience, it's usually possible to correct this for a child of any age, without surgery for a feeding tube. Don't leave this situation alone, and don't run to the endocrinologist for growth hormone injections— yet. A nutrition assessment should be completed first, with a registered dietitian or someone who knows child nutrition assessment and monitoring. Review total food intake carefully, and screen out bowel infections and inflammatory foods; these impede absorption of energy and nutrients, and diminish appetites, too. Have your pediatrician assess iron status and zinc status, two minerals that impact appetite (too little may diminish appetite). If you are giving your child supplements (including cod liver oil) with more than

5000 international units of vitamin A per day, stop (too much may lessen appetite).

Growth impairment. A "growth impairment" means your child has dropped fifteen or more percentage points off her previous place on the growth chart, for height or for weight. For example, if your child was at the 75th percentile for weight, then fell to the 60th, this is a growth impairment that warrants investigation. It doesn't matter that your child is still in the middle of the chart. It means your child may have stopped growing as she was genetically intended to grow. A growth impairment requires exploring in the context of your child's whole picture. Have there been changes in food intakes or eliminations? Recent illness or infections? New and considerable stressors, such as a move, divorce, or changes in how your child is able to eat at school? Is there a food allergy? I take all these into consideration when troubleshooting growth impairments. I also do a careful tally of food intake, to assess whether the child is actually eating enough or not.

Overweight. Children are clinically "overweight" when body mass index is at or above the 85th percentile for age. When they are above the 95th percentile BMI for age, they are clinically "obese." Either scenario warrants attention. If a child is gaining weight but not growing taller, this will skew the BMI toward "overweight." This does not necessarily mean the child needs to lose weight; it can mean that there is a food allergy, a gluten intolerance, or an inadequate total protein intake that is robbing the child of expected progress for stature (that is, leaving them shorter than expected for their weight). A child who is topping off the chart at the high end for both height and weight (big, tall, and fat) may have some untreated bowel infections driving a ravenous appetite for starchy empty calories, or may need some help tapping a good exercise plan.

How do you treat growth problems in children? Over my decade in practice, I've observed a blind spot on this in the pediatric medical community. Rather than work with underlying causes, there is a tendency among pediatricians to medicate the peripheral problems that go with growth impairments: laxatives for constipation, growth hormone injections for growth regression or growth failure, appetite stimulants (such as a drug called Periactin) for weak eating patterns, antidepressants or psych meds for overweight or obese children, allergy and asthma drugs for inflammation even when it's triggered by foods. Referrals for professional nutrition care are rare. The underlying problems are missed, and many kids don't get better—they get sicker, with more physical and emotional complications. Fortunately, nutrition care is a reliable, effective, evidence-based way to make your child feel, grow, and function better. Here's a checklist of considerations that your pediatrician may or may not know much about. If your doctor doesn't know, keep digging; remember, he hasn't been required to study nutrition in much depth or apply it in practice, so don't be intimidated. Search for the info you want, read up on it, and bring in your questions to your child's care visits.

Food allergy and sensitivity. Frequently throughout this book, I mention the impact of inflammation from foods, and how to screen for this. Skin scratch tests and IgE blood tests won't tell the whole story; they can miss gluten sensitivity, which can interfere with growth and with uptake of many nutrients, especially iron and other minerals. Children with food allergies tend to have lower total nutrient intakes and lesser growth patterns than kids without allergies. If your child's growth pattern seems to be lagging, ask for screening for both IgE and IgG food antibody responses to all major proteins your child eats.

Toxicity. Lead toxicity can interfere with appetite, so it's worth mentioning when looking at growth problems. Lead is poisonous, and it displaces minerals we need, such as iron and zinc. Children in marginal iron status will absorb more lead, given the same exposure, than children in healthy iron status. Surveillance data shows that most U.S. children have some low-level lead exposure. Since lead is fairly ubiquitous in our environment, this is yet another reason to make sure your child's iron status is good. It can, to some extent, protect against more lead uptake.

We may be hearing more about lead and toxicity in general. From heavy metals to weird plastics, parents are more aware of and concerned about what is going into our babies' bodies. Some rather shocking research has found that babies are now born with dozens of known carcinogens and toxins already in their placental cord blood. The CDC is undertaking a project called the National Children's Study to follow thousands of parent-baby pairs over the next twenty years, to see what toxins do what as children grow and develop. Curiously, though many parents and researchers have expressed concern about toxins in vaccines, this study won't include a vaccine-free cohort. It *will* include careful monitoring of lead levels.

If you want your child's lead level checked (your pediatrician may have done this already), you may have to look past blood, which may only show partial evidence of lead exposures. Lead in the body has a strong affinity for fatty tissues, such as brain, nerve, kidney, or liver, and it accumulates with repeat exposures. That means that a low level of lead in blood isn't necessarily reassuring: If there is some in blood, there may be more in your child's organ tissues. For the same reason, looking in blood for mercury is of little value, as it behaves in a similar fashion. Some complementary medicine providers use a test that looks for these metals in red blood cells rather than serum or whole blood. Another way to assess stored lead is to use a "provoking agent," that is, a substance that binds the stored lead into a form we can excrete; what is excreted is then measured in collected urine, or sometimes stool. Still other providers will take hair samples to test for heavy metals. But it has been demonstrated by a handful of researchers that children with autism do not show mercury in hair, while typical children do—implying that the children with autism may be unable to excrete it. For at least some children, using hair as a means to assess heavy metal exposures may mean little.

Over the last four decades, the CDC has repeatedly lowered what it defines as a tolerable lead level in children. Basically, there isn't one. Lead is negatively associated with IQ—that is, the more lead you are exposed to early in life, the lower your IQ will be. It is also associated with many neurodevelopmental problems. Even very low levels of lead in a child's blood correlate with cognitive and neurological impairments (not to mention appetite, metabolic, and nutrition problems). Because lead is so potentially injurious to the brain, the FDA previously approved chelation therapy to remove lead in children with a compound called DMSA (dimercaptosuccinic acid). In 2009, it abruptly pulled its approval for this tool, after DMSA was deemed acceptable for some fifteen years as a suitable treatment for lead toxicity in children. Some attribute this backpedaling to findings from the autism community, which showed that DMSA also safely removes mercury, the metal in question as a trigger for neurodevelopmental injury that is present in several vaccines. Endorsing a treatment for lead removal that also works for mercury would be tantamount to admitting that mercury should probably not be in vaccines in the first place, so the FDA has painted itself into quite a corner with this one. If even tiny amounts of lead are known triggers of neurodevelopmental problems, mercury becomes problematic, too, since it is known to be an even more potent neurotoxin than lead.

Instead, the CDC and American Academy of Pediatrics are gingerly acknowledging toxicity of heavy metals in children by focusing on lead screening and exposure prevention, but not on treatment, and not on mercury. We all harbor some heavy toxic metals, including mercury and lead. Infants and children are extremely vulnerable to these exposures because they are smaller than adults, and they are exposed to more of these now than most of their parents were early in life, owing to increased environmental pollutants and more vaccinations. Some special-needs children may be even more vulnerable, as suggested by clinical trials that have illustrated a diminished capacity to safely excrete toxic metals, compared to typical peers.

In any case, children with intractable growth impairments can be screened for heavy metal toxicity in a variety of ways. Lead, mercury, cadmium, or other toxic heavy metals may impair appetite, diminish enzyme function in the intestine, interfere with normal nutrient absorption, impede growth, and will disturb many metabolic pathways. You can:

- Have your pediatrician do a lead screening, as is currently recommended by the American Academy of Pediatrics.

- Consider a urine porphyrin test. This test looks at a group of metabolic compounds made by the body called porphyrins. Porphyrins may be elevated by heavy metal exposures, or when the body stores excess copper, a mineral we need in minute amounts for normal red blood cells and other functions. If your child's porphyrins are too high, many providers in the complementary medicine community suggest a chelation therapy for this, to help your child excrete these safely, or to balance copper, which can become a neurotoxin as well if too much is stored in tissues or circulating in the wrong form. See the resources section for labs that offer this test, if your doctor isn't familiar with it.

- Avoid mercury and lead exposures. Exposures occur with flu shots, some routine childhood vaccinations, some paints, agricultural and industrial chemicals, some toys, kids' jewelry, and common consumer products. Check a site called TheSoftLanding.com for toxin-free products for babies and kids.

- Talk to a licensed naturopathic doctor (ND) about options to safely remove toxic heavy metals stored in your child's body, if you have concerns that this is a problem. Methods range from using DMSA, to oral supplements of herbal tools such as chlorophyll and curcumin, to topical or oral glutathione products, or other supplements such as certain amino acid blends with minerals, N-acetyl cysteine, or alpha lipoic acid. Chelation protocols usually use tools that boost our native chemistry—that is, compounds we normally make in our own cells to excrete heavy metals are given as supplements, along with a provoking agent such as DMSA. Many protocols exist, and have good safety records. EDTA (calcium di-sodium EDTA) has been used as well, but this has had more safety concerns compared to other tools. One death occurred in a child infused with the wrong type of EDTA, a physician error. Chelation should be done with a knowledgeable provider with specific training in this area of practice. Since essential metals such as iron, zinc, selenium, and others can be depleted by chelating agents, it is important to work with a trained professional.

Bowel infections. Here I go again, bringing up bowel infections! But these truly are a cornerstone for so much in children. From setting up normal immune signaling in infancy to affecting behavior in children with autism, there is a much bigger role for these in health and disease than is currently appreciated. Growth patterns are linked to bowel flora, too, whether we are talking babies or big kids. When appetites are narrow, picky, self-limited to a very few foods, or ravenous for starchy sweets, it's time to assess what is going on in your child's bowel flora forest. From previously potty-trained kids with stool incontinence, to kids with reflux that won't quit, to others with a diet of pasta and butter only—these simply aren't healthy patterns for a child. Nutrients are lacking here, or being malabsorbed. Adjust bowel flora to its healthiest. Once restored, healthy bowel flora will help your child's appetite broaden, sugary cravings may quit, and more nutrients can be absorbed.

Use a stool microbiology test to check for overgrowths of fungal strains (candida, saccharomyces, or rhodotorula) or unwanted bacteria (certain enterobacter strains, klebsiella strains, campylobacter, clostridia, strep strains, and more). Treat these if they are out of whack. Using low-dose probiotics (less than 10 billion CFUs per day) won't do much good in a child with years of yeast infections in the gut. You may need a potent herbal antifungal

drop, such as citrus seed extract, uva ursi, Biocidin drops (a blend of strong antifungal, antimicrobial herbs), or a curcumin supplement (one called Enhansa is particularly promising). When choosing which ones to use, consider what your child's stool sensitivity panel says are effective agents, what he is capable of swallowing (drops, liquids, powders, capsules), what medications he is on, and what foods or herbs are known allergens for him. Other common antifungal herbs and supplements:

- Oil of oregano (capsules or used topically, diluted in vegetable oil)

- Cranberry extract (pills or capsules)

- Caprylic acid (capsules; this is a derivative of coconut oil)

- Undecylenic acid (capsules)

- Garlic extracts or certain chemicals in garlic, such as ajoene

- Tea tree oil (used topically)

- Black walnut hull or husk extract (tincture or drops)

- Goldenseal and other herbs containing berberine (tinctures)

- Berberine (capsules)

- Pau d'arco

- Turmeric (used both topically and as capsules)

These all have excellent safety records when used properly, but you should seek guidance with a licensed health care provider who is experienced and trained in herbs for kids before giving

them to your child. Naturopathic doctors do exactly that—*they train in the use of nonprescription agents such as nutrients and herbs*—so don't be surprised if your mainstream MD resources are not up to speed for answering these questions. I have found that pediatricians are often unfamiliar with the extent of the negative impact fungal infections can have on children, and may not be accustomed to prescribing for this. In that case, herbs work well, and sometimes better, than the medication could. Probiotics help, too, but children will need high doses (more than 12–15 billion CFUs per day) of the right strains for several weeks or months before a fungal infection may disappear. For this reason, I usually like to check with my clients' pediatricians to see if they will allow the antifungal medication, or use herbs to directly kill the fungal infection. Following these with the right probiotics usually does the trick.

Doctor's Data stool microbiology panels include a sensitivity panel to show what agents—herbal and prescription—effectively killed found species on your sample. This takes the guesswork out of how to treat a bowel infection. Doing this has reliably reversed wasting and growth failure in a number of children in my practice. It has also helped overweight children normalize their weight-to-height ratios and eat a better total diet.

What if your doctor is simply not on board with this strategy? See if you can work with another provider who is more open to these complementary medicine treatments. You can also use web-based services such as DirectLabs.com to get this type of testing done. An MD consult on your lab findings is typically included in the fee for the test, or available as an add-on. Stool microbiology testing is relatively inexpensive; it currently costs about $85–$90 to get this test done.

Mineralize. As mentioned already, low zinc and iron stores can diminish appetites in children, besides triggering myriad nutrition problems. These minerals are plentiful in meat, pork, lamb, shellfish, almonds, cashews, sunflower seeds, chickpeas, molasses, and black beans. An ordinary supplement dose is 15–30 milligrams per day for zinc, and 5 milligrams per day for iron, unless your child's circumstances warrant different dosing. Lab work plus signs and symptoms can identify what your child needs. Signs of low zinc status include white dots on nails, teeth grinding, mouthing objects and chewing on nonfood items (in kids past this stage developmentally), acne, delayed onset for puberty, growth failure, frequent infections, or slow-to-heal cuts and scrapes. Low iron status signs are pallor, irritability, lethargy, hyperactivity, frequent infections, translucent-looking skin, insomnia, or inattention.

Sneaky tactics. A bumper crop of cookbooks are available to help parents hide vegetables and fruits in foods their kids already like. Pumpkin or butternut puree in sweet breads or pancakes, minced vegetables in meatballs, carrot juice or spinach in smoothies, or zucchini in cookies is all well and good. As long as you are not unhappily chained to your stove, there isn't more sugar than veggies in these foods, and your child is managing some new servings of fruits and vegetables daily, dive in. That said, if this is the only way your child will accept some fruits and vegetables, then there is some work to do. A willingness to eat a variety of foods is a sign that your child's nutrition status, digestion, and bowel flora are returning to normal. It may be *common*, but it isn't *normal* for children to self-restrict to three or four foods, or throw tantrums at age eight if pasta and butter aren't on the menu every evening. Treating bowel infections and replenishing minerals with a good supplement can help pull your child's food intake back toward more variety. You shouldn't have to stick your landings every day with culinary gymnastics to get your child to eat an asparagus tip! Your child should be open to trying the asparagus, and usually will be once she is physically comfortable digesting most foods.

The same goes for sneaky tactics to add calories. Don't rely on inflammatory dairy foods to do this. If you have used supports such as Peptamen Junior, Boost, Ensure, whole milk, ice cream, whole yogurt, and lots of cheese with marginal success for repairing your child's growth pattern, check your child's IgE *and* IgG to casein and whey (dairy proteins). If they are elevated, your child's immune system is reacting to these, so relying on calories that include lots of dairy will backfire. An irritable, loose, or constipated stool pattern can signal inflammation from a food protein, as do chronic colds and infections, congestion, bloating, or picky eating habits. Switch to something such as So Delicious brand coconut milk (now sold in cartons like regular milk). This is high calorie, but low protein, so you will need to add a protein source. Try SHS North America Essential Amino Acid Mix (these are medical-grade amino acids used in tube feedings), Kirkman Amino Support Powder (a much cheaper supplement that is flavored, with a few other amines added beyond the essential ones), or Ultracare for Kids from Metagenics (rice protein augmented with essential lysine, plus calories, some fats, and vitamins and minerals). Never mind adding soy protein daily, unless you are certain it is not problematic for your child. Rule out inflammation from other major proteins, too—soy, gluten, egg, and nuts at the very least—if your child is struggling with any growth impairment.

What about calcium if you withdraw dairy foods? This is easy to replace. Calcium supplements abound. Some protein powders and amino acid supplements already contain calcium at levels similar to milk. For example, if your child likes Ultracare for Kids supplemental powder in juice or smoothies daily, notice that it contains 250 milligrams of calcium carbonate per scoop. This adds up fast—don't overload your child with calcium. In total, 800–1000 milligrams of calcium per day are enough, especially if your child is also willing to eat some calcium-rich nondairy foods, such as broccoli, tofu, bok choy, kale, temper, sesame thins, molasses, fortified juices, or almonds. If you want to use a chewable supplement, remember that many of these contain dairy flavorings and are usually calcium carbonate, a form best taken with food. Calcium carbonate is the ingredient in chewable antacids (such as TUMS) that buffer stomach acid, which may actually worsen your child's digestion, absorption, and growth pattern over time. Other forms of calcium might work better, depending on your child's circumstances. See "Reflux and Poor Growth," below.

Tube Feedings and Modular Feeding

Children on tube feedings may gain weight better, have less mucus in the tube, experience less spit-up and vomiting, or move their bowels more regularly when an easy-to-absorb food source is used in the tube. It's surprising how often I encounter children who are tube fed with formulas or pureed items that are poorly tolerated or badly digested, which will only lead to more lackluster results, or more chronic illness. Some parents I work with successfully puree a regular diet, including fiber sources, and add it to the tube. Other children need specialized formulas in the tube. In either case, avoiding inflammatory trigger foods can make this go better. All the same tricks apply for tube-fed kids as for orally fed kids in this regard. Assess both IgE (allergy) and IgG (sensitivity) reactions in your child, and prioritize them. If many are positive, you can't withdraw them all. Pick the top two to four offenders and rotate the lesser ones. For kids who have used a casein-based tube feed but who end up showing inflammation from it, switch to elemental options such as Elecare or Neonate. These are available formulated for infants and for children over one year. Formulas such as Vivien, Ensure, or Peptamen Junior may fail for kids with dairy sensitivity. Other children may not tolerate even the elementals very well. They may struggle with the corn-based carbohydrate source, or with the aspartame and glutamine in these products. The amino acids can be problematic in children with a history of seizures. In these cases, I turn to modular feeding.

Modular feeding simply means compounding a formula from separate ingredients that a child may tolerate well, when a prepared commercial option doesn't exist. I have done this for some children in my practice; I've also encountered parents taking this on without medical guidance, in a desperate attempt to find foods their children tolerate. Usually, good things come out of their efforts (smart parents!), and we find ways together to improve things even further. Modular feedings have to match your child's nutrition needs exactly, while avoiding other problems—such as inflammation, seizures, growth failure, overweight, constipation, and diarrhea. If you are creating your own formula, run it by your pediatrician or gastro MD to make sure you're getting it right.

- If it says "milk," it doesn't necessarily have the nutrients of cow's milk. Milks from rice, hemp, almond, oat, or hazelnut are poor sources of protein, calories, and fats. If you are using these as a major calorie and protein source in your tube feed, your child needs to augment his intake.

- Add eggs, meats, chicken, turkey, beans, or lentils for protein, if your child can tolerate these.

- Soy milk is hard for many children to tolerate, just like cow's milk. Use this option gingerly, preferably not daily, unless you are certain it isn't inflammatory and it works well for your child. Soy can be constipating, is high in oxalates (irritating for some children), and can diminish absorption of some nutrients such as iron.

- If several major food proteins trigger inflammation, consider free essential amino acids to replace poorly tolerated protein sources. Your doctor or a registered dietitian can authorize SHS North America Essential Amino Acid Mix as a protein source in modular feeding. Get their guidance on how much to add to the feed, and what other foods to add around it, for calories and fats and oils.

- Protein powders from rice, soy, egg, whey, or dairy may be helpful if you are certain your child tolerates them without inflammation. Rice protein is of poor value and must be augmented with an amino acid called lysine, or with foods that contain lysine, such as beans or corn.

- Don't rely on vegan alternate milks as infant formula. For many reasons, they are not nutritionally adequate or appropriate for a baby.

- Consider So Delicious brand coconut milk as a base for modular feeding. It is rich in easy-to-digest fats, is fortified with some vitamins and minerals, and has only 80 calories in 8 ounces. This can work for overweight tube-fed children who can't get the physical activity they need. You will need to add a protein source to this product. For underweight children, add calories from medium chain triglycerides, oils you know your child can digest, or easy-to-manage carbohydrates such as winter squash, pumpkin puree, or Wax Orchards brand pure fruit sweetener (this has no added sugar or corn syrup, which can be too challenging for some children to digest).

- One more option I have used in modular feedings when many other tools failed is goat milk. Powdered goat milk can be reconstituted and blended into a formula, with additional modular calories or nutrients as needed. Digestive enzymes for lactose, casein, and mucus (with a product called Mecosta) were added to this formula with success. Some children who are intolerant to cow's milk protein can manage goat milk protein well.

In each of these cases, the calories per ounce of formula were thoughtfully set based on the child's nutrition assessment, as were total protein, percentage of calories from fats and carbs, types of fats and carbs, and recommended ounces of formula daily. Each child is unique. Modular feeding can work well whether your child is tube fed or on oral feeding. It's best to get some professional guidance on this, so your child's nutrition needs can be correctly met.

Reflux and Poor Growth

Another drug class (besides psychotropic meds) that has spiked for use in children is reflux medications. More reflux medications are getting approved by the FDA for use in children; some were withdrawn after being deemed unsafe. Data on reflux meds for children suggests that these are probably overprescribed. That is, they are often given to infants and children who don't have too much acid in their stomachs. The only way to know for sure if your child's stomach is too acid is to do a pH probe test, which a gastroenterologist can do. But the test is invasive and impractical, so it's common for doctors simply to try the reflux medication instead. These are intended for a short time frame, perhaps a week or two, maybe up to eight weeks. But it's not unusual for me to encounter children using them for months or years, and it appears there are negative effects of altering stomach acid production for so long, especially during childhood when we are growing. Changing the acidity of the stomach and GI tract changes the absorption of nutrients. I have observed several cases in which long-term use of reflux medication may have triggered stunting and growth failure, owing to weakened digestion and weaker ability to eat enough food. Whether scenarios such as these are, in fact, due to long-term use of reflux meds will have to be examined in research. Meanwhile, my own clinical experience has prompted me to make alternative suggestions for clients.

It has also been argued that reflux medications may not treat the problem correctly in infants and children. They were designed to treat overacid production in adults. But in babies and kids, reflux can occur for other reasons—such as inflammation or allergy, bowel infections, normal spit-up, GI motility issues, or delayed coordination of suck-swallow-breath skills or chewing and swallowing skills. Reflux medications in these cases will certainly diminish the acidity of a child's stomach—but this is a slippery slope. The weaker the stomach's acid, the less digestion occurs. This means digestion isn't initiated as intended, and food sits idle in the stomach—causing more reflux. Hormones and enzymes that depend on the stomach's acidity to "turn on" stay off. The stomach empties its contents into the small intestine at the wrong pH, hormones and enzymes don't kick in to trigger normal digestion, and digestion progresses at a tepid pace. Meanwhile, fungal microbes such as candida thrive in the more buffered bowel environment. In my practice, I have repeatedly seen dependence on reflux medication add up to intestinal fungal infections; constipation; impactions; weak, picky appetites; and poor growth pattern. While it can be hard to convince the attending GI doctor to give it a try, using as strong an antifungal medication as can be allowed (like Diflucan or Flagyl) can sometimes resolve the reflux, constipation, and impactions. This can clear the path for healthier, more acid-producing species to populate the gut that help us digest food, and ultimately help normalize digestion and lessen reflux. If history, signs, symptoms, and stool culture indicate it, see if your physician will explore antifungal therapy.

Somehow, reflux medications caught on with the pediatric community in the 1990s as a quick-and-easy fix. Many youngsters do initially feel better on these medications. They can help ulcerations heal, if those are present in the esophagus, and if your child truly has gastroesophageal reflux disease from an overacid stomach. In that case, the right medication can resolve a great deal of pain, and this is especially pertinent for babies, and for children with autism, who can't tell you when they are in pain. Meanwhile, many children get little to no relief, or soon need to increase the dose of a reflux medication, only to end up topping out at the highest allowable dosage with reflux as bad as before. If your child has gotten stuck on a reflux medication, still has reflux, and is not growing as robustly as expected, you can:

- Use stool microbiology testing to rule out intestinal infections—and treat them.

- Double-check the stool microbiology with a urine organic acid test (OAT) for microbial acids, that is, acids produced only by certain microbes (not people). If the stool culture didn't adequately capture suspected microbial overgrowths, a urine microbial OAT can affirm whether or not detrimental microbes are there.

- Discuss the possibility of using a pH probe test or other measures with your doctor, to find out if your child truly needs the reflux medication. Work out a plan to wean off it with your doctor.

- Assess both IgE (allergy) and IgG (sensitivity) reactions in your child. Remove the top two or three offenders, and replace them with equally nutritious foods. Rotate other trigger foods. I have frequently witnessed just gluten withdrawal resolve reflux, in children who had elevated gliadin IgG antibody, even when they did not have celiac disease. Ask your doctor about checking antigliadin IgG antibody.

Children who vomit undigested food hours after eating when they aren't ill or have no fever, who say they are full when having eaten just a few bites, or who have used reflux medication for a long time may have stomachs that don't produce enough acid to normally begin the process of digesting food. If you are certain that the esophagus is healthy, try gently acidifying the stomach to improve digestion. A supplement called betaine hydrochloride is a common digestive aid. Try one capsule (about 200 milligrams) at the start of a meal. If no change and no complaints, give your child two. For children who can't swallow capsules, many naturopaths recommend giving a teaspoon of cider vinegar in a little water with a meal, and using it in the same way: Increase the amount if it seems to improve comfort, appetite, and digestion in your child. Some supplemental enzymes can help digestion even when the stomach and small intestine are not as acid as they should be. All of these tools can trigger pain when ulcers or inflamed tissue are present in the esophagus, so be sure this is not the case before trying them. Generally, since these are nonprescription ("natural") tools, naturopathic doctors will have more experience than MDs in how and when to use them—so don't be discouraged if your pediatrician isn't sure how to guide you. You can find a naturopath in your area by visiting Naturopathic .org and entering your zip code into the "find a doctor" feature.

Gentle herbal tinctures are available for young children as a means to stimulate the output of digestive hormones and enzymes. Typical ingredients in these preparations are peppermint, licorice root, ginger root, chamomile, cardamom, fennel, or rosemary, usually in a coconut glycerin (not alcohol) base. Stronger versions called "digestive bitters" can be taken ahead of meals to more potently stimulate digestion. WishGarden Herbs, Nature's Way, and

HerbPharm make these tinctures. Check with a naturopath to explore how to safely administer these to infants and children.

About food. Many kids I work with have been placed on special diets by their families or by other providers before I meet them, for a variety of reasons. More often than you might think, children who are growing poorly are stuck that way because their food intakes can't support normal growth. They actually do not eat enough. Incredibly, this übersimple part of the puzzle is frequently overlooked entirely. Children may be referred to an endocrinologist for complex blood work to search for that magic hormone deficit, before a dietitian evaluates their food intake and growth pattern. This is backward. Have food intakes evaluated first, and consider how physically busy and active your child is, too. This (obviously) will increase their caloric needs. And:

- For a child growing poorly who likes milk, yogurt confections, ice cream, cheese, and then more milk, well, adding still *more* dairy calories isn't going to help. It's likely that the dairy protein this child loves is malabsorbed. Assess IgE and IgG inflammation from milk and work up a different protein source if positive.

- For a child showing some unexpected regression for stature in the context of enough total calories (that is, progress for getting taller has slowed down, or dropped more than fifteen points), review gluten sensitivity. If even marginally positive, yank all gluten for a four-month period to see if growth (or reflux, mood, focus, irritability, odd stooling pattern) begins to correct. This is not hard to do these days, now that gluten-free foods are available in many stores and on the Internet.

I've often heard the old saw in pediatrics that says babies and kids will eat the amount of food they need, if you leave them to it and stop fussing over it. But for much of the population I work with, this is not true. Instead, eating becomes a dreaded chore that grinds the spirits of parents and kids alike. Children well into preschool years may eat only if fed by their parents' hands, even when their own hands seem to work just fine; others may eat only if distracted by certain TV shows or DVDs. Some work with therapists to map out strict behavior plans for eating. Still others need absolutely no interruptions or distractions, lest they pitch a nerve-singing tantrum and stop eating. Even babies can struggle with eating enough: Infants can lose so much of their feedings through chronic vomiting, spitting up, or having loose, wet stool (more than four per day on a regular basis) that they struggle to earn an ounce of weight. They also require so many more calories per pound than kids and adults do just to *be*, that lengthy crying jags become calorically very costly for them, if they happen every day for hours on end.

If this describes mealtimes in your household, nutrition assessment tools can help you target what to do. In my experience, these are kids who do need total food intakes reviewed, along with a look at activity level/energy output, inflammation trigger foods screened, and bowel infections identified and treated. Oral tactile defensiveness—in which children are inexplicably averse to putting food in their own mouths, or to all but one or two food textures—may diminish when inflammatory foods, especially gluten, are identified and removed, when minerals such as zinc are replenished, and when bowel infections and reflux are resolved.

This is such a common error that I must mention it again: Don't remove every food that pops up as positive on an allergy (IgE), sensitivity (IgG) panel, or other tests that suggest food intolerance or inflammation. This is simply unworkable for children, who must grow. They need enough high-value protein sources to do that, and they need adequate calories from fats and carbohydrates around that protein as well. High-value protein is protein that delivers all eight or ten essential amino acids, the ones we cannot manufacture ourselves. We have to eat them. If you have pulled soy, dairy, wheat, nuts, egg, lentils, beef, poultry, and beans out of your child's diet, then you've pulled out pretty much all viable protein sources. If you've also decided that every vegetable or fruit that was even moderately positive on that lab sheet has to go, too, you are definitely in doomed-to-fail territory. If your child has been diagnosed with multiple food allergies and significant intestinal inflammation (this can only be seen with endoscopy or pill camera), then your doctor should have prescribed an elemental formula such as Elecare or Neocate. These deliver free amino acids with carbs, fats and oils, and vitamins and minerals. Elemental formulas (also called amino acid–based formulas or AABF) have shown demonstrable benefit to gut tissue repair in children with Crohn's disease. They can actually help repair gut tissue—so use them if this is on your child's to-do list. Bottom line for multiple food protein allergy:

- Work with four major offenders at most, and rotate the rest.

- Use a supplement of oral liposomal glutathione. See why below.

- Use free amino acids in whatever form your child accepts and tolerates, either as a modular feed or in AABF.

- Support protein intake with adequate intakes of carbohydrates and fats and oils. This protects the protein so that it can be used for tasks such as tissue repair, instead of being burned for energy.

- Incorporate a long-term gut health regimen with probiotics, treating intestinal infections, or both.

My goal in managing multiple food allergies in kids, whether they have growth issues or not, is to repair gut wall tissue to the point where they can eat more foods with no ill effects. I haven't encountered many children who just "grew out of" a food allergy or intolerance. What I have found is that the baby who was colicky and miserable on cow's milk protein formulas may become the child with asthma, eczema, or stooling problems a few years later. Did they grow out of that milk protein issue, or did it just become a deeper problem? It's much easier to prevent these outcomes in school-age kids by redirecting all this in infancy and toddlerhood than it is to reverse it later on.

Glutathione: "The Mother of All Antioxidants"

That's what Mark Hyman, MD, functional medicine practitioner and author, calls this miraculous molecule. It has been the focus of hundreds of research publications because of its excellent capability to manage oxidative stress, which worsens all disease conditions, from Alzheimer's to autoimmune disorders. Though we make glutathione ourselves, our capacity to do so can be overwhelmed by toxic exposures, poor diet, liver damage, or malabsorption. Cells that stop making glutathione die. Along with the right probiotics, it's a favorite tool of mine to reverse and repair damage from years of inflammatory responses to a food protein. Glutathione is a molecule we make in our cells from amino acids. Volumes could be inserted here about its benefits and its importance in many chronic conditions, including autism (a condition in which depleted glutathione has been documented). But for our purposes at this moment, let's just say that it is our most important intracellular antioxidant. It stops reactive "oxygen species," or free radicals, from literally tearing cell chemistry apart. Where there is inflammation, there is impaired glutathione synthesis; in inflammatory bowel diseases, low glutathione manufacture has been documented in gut tissue. This is not good. This means that tissue damage can progress, without protective glutathione around to stop it. "Oxidative damage" is what glutathione prevents, and oxidative damage is a key concern in the progression of inflammatory bowel diseases. Consider this supplement for a child with Crohn's disease or any bowel inflammation, since it is known to be depleted in those conditions. It has no known toxicity, and its relevance in body chemistry has been reviewed for decades.

When I have suggested it anecdotally, I have been impressed with glutathione's results for children with multiple food protein allergies. Reports of improved stools, calmer demeanor, and more willingness to try new foods typically attend use of liposomal glutathione. Subjective stuff, and as usual, research here would help (so far, the research is strong for those with Alzheimer's who supplement glutathione, but there is little done on its role in mitigating food allergies or autoimmune disorders). But if parents and kids are happy, I'm happy. Use the liposomal form of this supplement—a liquid—rather than powders, so that the glutathione is delivered to intestinal wall tissue intact. This form encases the glutathione in bubbles of fatty molecules—liposomes—to enhance its delivery across gut tissue. Children who are depleted for glutathione and for sulfur chemistry in general (glutathione is a sulfur-rich molecule) may react to introducing it too quickly. They may become irritable, agitated, or wakeful. If this occurs in a child given glutathione, it can be confirming that they indeed need it, but must begin with very small doses—just a drop or two of liposomal glutathione to start. Glutathione supplementation may also trigger children with high oxalates to "dump" more oxalates via urine, and this can be agitating, too. In that case, it may be best to start with replenishing sulfur first with Epsom salts in nightly baths, and amino acids that are needed to make glutathione, such as N-acetyl cysteine. Once again, an experienced provider can help you navigate these nuances in lessening destructive oxidative stress for your child.

When It Comes to Food, Let Kids Be Kids—At Least Some of the Time

When looking at your child's food intake, don't apply adult rules. For example, many parents restrict carbohydrates and fats or oils in their kids' diets, believing that what is healthy for adults is healthy for kids. Not really true, especially for kids with any special needs. Kids need varied fats, oils, and carbohydrates. They don't need trans fats, hydrogenated fats, or a limited variety of fats from animal foods only. Incorporate variety for fats and oils with nuts, plants, and seed oils, too, to meet your child's needs for brain and nerve tissue, cholesterol and hormone production, healthy cell wall structures, and more. Children need cholesterol (we all do), especially at puberty. We can make our own, so it isn't terribly important to eat it—but it isn't harmful either, if your child has an overall balanced diet and good physical activity. I encourage the inclusion of organic, high omega-3 eggs when they are tolerated by kids, because these are full of so many good fats, protein, and some vitamins and minerals. Another favorite of mine is coconut milk, unsweetened and unadulterated, to add to curries, smoothies, or baked goods. Its shorter chain fats are easy to digest and absorb, compared to the long chains found in oils from corn or soy. Ghee, which is butter with all dairy solids removed, is a great option, too, especially if your child misses the taste of butter but can't use it due to milk protein allergy, or if you need a stiff fat for baking things such as pie crusts or cookies. Avocado, flax meal or oil, sesame tahini, almond butter, olive oil, sunflower seeds, or any tolerated nuts themselves are healthy additions you should allow for your child. Fats and oils should comprise about a third of your child's total calories, under most circumstances. Overweight children can limit these if necessary to some extent, but they, too, still need a variety of healthy fats and oils for normal structure and function in cells and tissues.

Though we've all learned to look askance at cholesterol, it is an important molecule. It provides the base structure for sex hormones, is crucial for cell wall structure and function, helps neurons connect and repair while we sleep, and helps us digest other fats. Interestingly, in some children with autism, exceedingly low cholesterol levels have been found. Genetic defects that alter cholesterol metabolism were ruled out, so why it was too low was unclear. But this will be the case in a child when body mass index is too low, when a child is too thin, or when total fat and calorie intakes are too low—all of which I have repeatedly found in children with autism. You don't have to take cholesterol supplements to repair this (you can if you like), but simply eating more total fats from all sources, as well as more carbohydrate calories, will help your body make more of its own cholesterol. Besides all the jobs cholesterol has, it is apparently important to maintain a normal level for another reason: Research over the last three decades has illustrated that when total cholesterol is low, behavior may change for the worse. Suicidality, aggressive behavior, violent behavior, and even criminality have been linked to depressed cholesterol levels. Also linked with this is the finding that cholesterol and testosterone are inversely related: If cholesterol is depressed, testosterone may be driven up, and this is suspected of triggering behavior issues.

Overrestricting calories from carbohydrates is problematic, too. Raw foods, fermented foods, and yeast-free diets have grown in popularity, especially in the autism community. Intakes that rely mostly on those foods tend to be too low in total calories for children. They aren't calorically dense enough to support normal growth or optimal assimilation of proteins. You may have heard that Americans eat more protein than they need, and this is often true for adults or kids with regular diets and no special needs. But if your child is managing a restricted diet for any reason, has a growth impairment, or has an inflammatory condition, you will want to maximize the right distribution of amino acids for tissue repair and chemical construction (hormones, glutathione, neurotransmitters, our own proteins, etc.). If your child's food intake is scant, protein is what you are asking them to burn for energy. This is an inefficient process that requires extra work by liver and kidney tissues, which are called into duty to extract the carbon skeletons out of the protein and waste the nitrogen into urine. Instead of botching this chemistry, you can:

- Permit a rotation of *some* fermented and raw foods if your child likes them, but don't rely on these for major calories or dietary bulk.

- Allow about two-thirds of your child's total intake to be tolerable, healthy carbs. What those are may vary for children, but consider items allowed on the Specific Carbohydrate Diet, which are most easily digested. You can see these at PecanBread.com. There are dozens of carb-dense fruits and vegetables on this list, along with recipes at the site.

- Don't avoid food to treat bowel infections or gut dysbiosis. This often backfires into an overrestricted, calorically depleted diet for children. If bowel flora is this bad, treat with a medication, the right probiotics, or targeted antimicrobial herbs.

- If you've withdrawn gluten, switch in everything gluten-free, including bread, pasta, bagels, corn tortillas if tolerated, corn, sweet potato, quinoa, black rice (also called "forbidden rice," this is a purplish black variety that is rich in iron and has a nutty flavor), or whole grain brown rice. Learn about alternative flours made out of rice, potato, tapioca, beans, and so on, so you can cook and bake most all the same things as before.

- Pick up a copy of *The Gluten-Free Italian Cookbook* by Mary Capone (a celiac with an authentic Italian culinary and family heritage), Bette Hagman's *Gluten-Free Gourmet* cookbooks, or Rebecca Reilly's *Gluten-Free Baking* for special-occasion baked treats. These are just a few of the many excellent resources out there, if you must withdraw gluten.

Normalizing both food intakes and food absorption is the key to normalizing growth pattern. Even growth hormone injections may not help as much as these two foundation pieces. Once your child's growth pattern is restored, many other things can go better, from infection fighting, to sleeping and playing, to focusing and behaving, and to simply eliminating toxins every day in stool, as we are meant to do. It's a reasonable goal to expect your child to be weaned off a tube and return to oral feeding, if oral skills and structures for feeding are intact. It's fair enough to want some freedom at mealtime, so you don't have to hand-feed your little bird yourself for years on end. Your child deserves the social context of food that you grew up enjoying, so it's reasonable to see if you can relax some of those dietary restrictions. Restoring an expected growth pattern can in itself go a long way toward supporting mood, preventing mood swings, and lessening anxiety in children. For targeted helps along those lines, see the next chapter.

Special Situations: Down's Syndrome and Mitochondrial Disorders

I mention these two conditions together since they overlap in regard to muscle tone and energy level, which tend to affect children who have Down's or "mito" disorders. Down's children also tend to show differences for growth pattern, compared to typical peers. Focus and attention can challenge these children, just by virtue of their having low energy and low affect much of the time. When I have had the opportunity to work with these children, the same nutrition screenings apply as for any other child in my practice. We rule out food sensitivities, especially from gluten (with an antigliadin IgG antibody test), we check for bowel infections, and we review critical nutrients that are often depleted, such as zinc, iron, or other minerals. We work in natural supports for easy stooling, as these kids may tend toward constipation—products such as FruitEze (a natural fruit concentrate), OxyPowder (a magnesium source), or vitamin C at multigram doses rather than milligrams.* And as always, a careful food diary tells me exactly what the child is eating, and whether his current intake is appropriate to support expected growth, functioning, and energy level.

But for Down's and mito kids, it may be fruitful to take it a little further. These conditions may warrant additional supports to improve their cells' capacity to produce energy. One key for this is an amino acid called carnitine, which transfers certain fatty acid molecules into cell structures called mitochondria. Mitochondria are like your cells' power plants—they produce energy. Anything that disrupts carnitine's function or availability can create features of carnitine deficiency, which range widely—from low tone and low affect to heart failure. Carnitine deficiency will

---

* The same advice applies for checking with a provider before using high doses of nutrients for constipation. More strategies for resolving constipation can be found on Talk About Curing Autism's (TACA) infamous "Poop Page" at Talk AboutCuringAutism.org.

keep muscles from working properly, and variants of this will affect smooth muscles (as in the heart or gastrointestinal tract) or skeletal muscles. A metabolic specialist MD can discern if your child has carnitine deficiency, and what type. Ask for a referral to a pediatric mitochondrial or metabolic specialist MD if your child has Down's syndrome or chronic low muscle tone. Children with carnitine deficiency will have trouble shifting from glucose to ketones for energy, which normally happens once we use up glucose derived from a recent meal or from stored sources. For this reason, when I encounter children who tolerate fasting periods especially badly—that is, they become exceedingly lethargic without snacks and meals at close intervals—screening for carnitine deficiency might be added to screening for blood sugar control. Fasting hypoglycemia (lower than normal blood sugar after an overnight fast) is common with carnitine deficiency, so it is important to correctly discern both pieces in children with this presentation. A pediatric occupational or physical therapist can diagnose problems with muscle tone for you, while the MD specialist can work up the lab data needed to sort out which metabolic issues to pursue.

Supplemental carnitine has shown mixed results—some positive, some neutral—in clinical trials for persons with Down's syndrome and mitochondrial disorders, not to mention Alzheimer's, migraines, heart disease, autism, and other conditions. Though it is not yet a standard procedure to screen children with autism for carnitine deficiency, research has found that they may tend to have significantly lower carnitine levels than normal. This may be a factor in sudden cardiac arrest that has tragically felled some children with autism. Other research suggests that carnitine deficiency may be a trigger for poor gut motility, meaning it may contribute to constipation unless carnitine is replenished. Carnitine is ample in meats, but can still be depleted in diets that include meats if carnitine transport mechanisms are flawed. It may be depleted in vegetarian diets or in protein malnutrition, too. When supplemented, carnitine is typically replenished orally along with its necessary cofactors: high-potency B-group vitamins, vitamin E, coenzyme Q10, and zinc, for starters. When used as a therapeutic measure, carnitine is given at doses of 100 milligrams per kilogram, as often as three times a day. These amounts need a medical rationale that a specialist can investigate for your child. Doses for children should not exceed 3 grams daily, and typically begin at 50 milligrams per kilogram per day.

With Nutrition-Focused Tools, Hope Is Always There

Don't presume that a special-needs child who has an inherited disorder can't improve. Children with Down's syndrome in my practice have exceeded the expectations of their parents, doctors, and teachers with leaps in progress for growth, academic performance, age-appropriate socialization, and energy, when given the opportunity to use nutrition-focused tools effectively. Be sure to at least rule out gluten sensitivity with a gliadin antibody test (not a celiac panel), and rule out zinc insufficiency as well. These are two nutrition pieces that reliably interfere with progression for stature (height), if they are problematic for a child.

Chapter Five

Special Needs at School

ATTENTION, FOCUS, LEARNING, BEHAVIOR,
DEPRESSION, AND ANXIETY

It's hard to remember how dramatically different the lives of children are now than they were just thirty years ago. Being without instant communication and virtually infinite information access is utterly inconceivable to young adults and children today. Whether it's using a web interface a teacher has set up for homework assignments, playing virtual games with unseen opponents via the Internet, or texting a friend in shorthand, children are now in a world where they must manage everything faster, sooner, better. Even CDs and videos, once astonishing for their novelty but now dinosaurs, were nonexistent. Before 1980, kids were less structured in their time, less scheduled, less pressured to perform on all fronts from athletics to academics at younger and younger ages; outdoors more, in front of screens less. The capacity to literally process what is going on around them—a brain-body skill that builds and integrates gradually throughout childhood and adolescence—was permitted to evolve. It arguably no longer is—and the child with special needs is the one who may suffer most in this scenario. Why? Because developmental and learning differences often involve some impairment in processing speed in the brain. Processing speed is critical for learning and for acquiring independence. For children with autism, processing all kinds of information and sensory inputs can be impaired at once; for a child with dyslexia, it may only be visual processing that is affected. In either case, learning, social, and most any other environments are harder for these children to manage.

Children with challenges such as autism spectrum disorders, ADHD or ADD, depression, anxiety, insomnia, or dyslexia are often baffled when it comes to knowing what the teacher just said, what the words on the page mean, how to fit in with a group of peers, or where their pencil went. Being lost like this while their peers are calmly processing the world around them and making progress can create even more anxiety and more of a sense of failure in these children. As the world moves faster and the demands on children have shifted from ordinary to crushing, parents face the hard choice of pharmaceutically altering a child's brain chemistry to meet the challenges of the changing world, or altering the child's world so she can evolve at her own pace—say, by dropping out of sight to raise children on a bucolic farm somewhere. Both choices are extremes fraught with disadvantages. Not only do entire educational philosophies rest on this point, but so do intense debates about what children need for health care, discipline, parenting, and daily routines.

Somewhere in between is a reasonable goal for the child, who needs to adapt to some degree to function in the world, and may need *some* help with brain chemistry to do that. There are nutrition-focused tools to help you find this balance. It is important to consider options like this because the safety, efficacy, ethics, and necessity of medicating children—to woefully understate it—is an ongoing question. A stark shift between today and 1980 is that millions of children now routinely take drugs to control behavior, mood, and attention, and this is no longer regarded as alarming. Many of these drugs are prescribed by pediatricians who admit to lacking adequate training to manage problems such as childhood depression, anxiety, or learning problems. It is frequently a child's pediatrician, and not a specialist in pediatric neurology, psychiatry, or psychology, that prescribes these medications. In fact, a letter by Claudia Gold, MD, published in the *New York Times* on May 7, 2010, stated that pediatricians may prescribe a medication for ADHD based on a single thirty-minute visit with one parent, and monitor only once every few months. While children appropriately and expertly diagnosed with something such as ADHD or generalized anxiety disorder can benefit from thoughtful prescribing, many do not. I wish I could quote data here to say that, on balance, emphatically, these drugs consistently succeed more than they fail in children. No research can say this; even if it did, I would still suggest that parents review nutrition supports before trying prescription medications. If for no other reason, it's important to remember that nutrition problems can profoundly interfere with learning, mood, sleep, and behavior in children—and psychotropic medications do not fix nutrition problems. It makes good clinical sense to rule out the easy stuff first.

Making this all the more confusing for everybody, including your doctor, is that the FDA allows pharmaceutical companies to market medications directly to children and parents. Ads for psychotropic medications splash across the web, children's TV shows, parenting magazines, and medical journals. Many have wondered how neutral scientific journals can be when they rely so heavily on pharmaceutical industry revenue. One study found that advertising by pharmaceutical companies in medical journals caused bias against nondrug therapies. The study reviewed eleven influential and highly lauded publications, including the *New England Journal of Medicine* and the *Journal of the American Medical Association*—the very publications your doctor probably turns to for guidance in practice. This leaves information on nondrug therapies not only harder to find, but harder to fund and publish.

Plenty of data exists to illustrate concern for the use of psychoactive drugs in children, drugs prescribed at ages as young as two years old. Nearly 600,000 reactions to medications occur each year in children. Are supplements safer? In 2008, the American Association of Poison Control Centers reported 1,315 deaths from medications, and none from supplements. Stimulants such as Ritalin, Adderall, and Concerta have been questioned for their link to sudden deaths and suicides in children as young as eleven years old who had no prior history of suicidality. Prescribing to children has risen steadily and dramatically since the days before videos and CDs. In the 1990s, double-digit percentage increases in prescribing these drugs occurred across continents, from the United Kingdom to the United States. No quarter was given even for preschool children, who received more stimulant medication than all other types of psychotropic medications combined. The long-term effects of medicating toddlers and preschoolers are unstudied. A recent study reviewing records of nearly 35,000 children in the UK using psychotropic medications (incredible in itself that this large a study group was not hard to find) found that *all* had been given an *average* of at least four of these; that once again, more prescriptions for stimulants such as Ritalin were given than any other drug; and that stimulant prescriptions rose nearly a hundredfold in the last half of the 1990s. Boys got more stimulants than girls; girls got more antidepressants.

Studies such as these usually include a comment in the abstract reminding us that these drugs are often prescribed for children even though they have not been licensed for use in that age group, that they are prescribed for conditions for which they are not approved, or that there is not sufficient data to know whether these prescribing practices are truly safe. Authors of these research articles usually conclude their abstracts with a call for caution, more safety studies, or some measure of restraint around prescribing for children. But where is this to be found? Until providers learn to work beyond their prescription pads, little will change.

Learning about the pharm-free options that maximize nutrition is one way to go. It's prudent to work with nutrition-focused tools for kids struggling with anxiety, attention or focus concerns, hyperactivity, depression, mood swings, or reactivity, because it's safe, it's cheap, and psych meds can't fix nutrition deficits that may trigger or worsen these problems. But it can be hard to adjust to the reality that nutrition rarely offers that one magic bullet, which is exactly how we are conditioned to think about using medications for these problems. Yes, I have observed children's behavior, countenance, and lives change dramatically with nutrition tools—but in each case, parents were ready to let go of the idea that nutrition care should work like a single prescription pill given daily. When nutrition problems are bad enough to trigger what looks like behavior problems, they have typically been entrenched a long while, leaving cells and metabolic pathways bereft of nutrients they need to operate optimally. Some nutrients can be quickly replenished; other corrections take weeks or months to set in for the child, especially when there are growth delays, chronic inflammation, or depleted stores of nutrients such as iron, essential fats, or vitamin D. Any functions directly or distantly dependent on nutrients can take time to come back online.

Your Key Tools for School

Before your child is given a medication to function better in a school environment, make sure that some baseline nutrition pieces are intact first. When these are not intact, ample data on child nutrition over several decades suggests that learning, focus, behavior, and cognition may be affected. Any child, special needs or not, will struggle more to focus, behave, concentrate, and stay organized when these things are off-kilter. Burdening a special-needs child even further with these nutrition deficits is like swimming upstream. Plug in these basics to help your child's brain and body go with, rather than against, the flow.

Check iron status. Normal iron status is critical for learning. Anemia is the result of entrenched iron deficiency; having anemia in infancy and early childhood is linked to long-term impairments in IQ, cognition, psychomotor skills, and even the likelihood of finishing school. We can have poor iron status without frank anemia—this is iron depletion, something that is not unusual to find in my own practice. Either scenario may depress our capacity to make enough red blood cells to carry oxygen, which of course the brain needs to do anything and everything. Both poor iron status and anemia have been linked to problems with learning and performing math concepts and tasks, as well as problems with focus, cognition, mood, and irritability in children. Throughout childhood, normal iron status is necessary for normal development, learning, and immune function, not to mention breathing! Signs of weak iron status include pallor, shiners at eyes, cold hands and feet, insomnia, brittle nails, and ultimately, shortness of breath and fatigue and lassitude. A classic red flag for iron deficiency in children is a desire to eat nonfood items such as dirt, ice, sand, or other unusual substances. This is not as rare as you might think: One child entered my office and promptly removed his shoes to lick the ice and sand out of the treads, to which his mother commented, "He always does that." A child who is determined to chew and devour pencils (or their erasers) should probably be screened for iron status, and other minerals as well, such as zinc, magnesium, selenium, chromium, and calcium. Since iron is toxic when dosed incorrectly, don't add it without professional guidance (see below).

Paradoxically, children in marginal iron status may not look lethargic—they can display quite a bit of vigor being crabby! Iron is a marginal nutrient for many children in the United States, and it remains a priority public health issue here. Special-needs children who have inflammation, poor diet, celiac disease, Crohn's disease, or chronic malabsorption for any reason may be at risk for impaired iron status. More discussion on this is in Chapter 3. If there is any question about iron for your child, talk to your doctor. Your pediatrician should check:

- Hemoglobin (Hgb)

- Hematocrit (Hct)

- Ferritin

- Total iron binding capacity (TIBC)

- Complete blood count (CBC), which checks the number and types of red blood cells

Note: Iron supplements should not be used without professional supervision. Iron is toxic if given in the wrong dose, so check with your doctor before you give any iron preparations to your child. If iron supplementation is called for, many doctors will prescribe a high daily dose of ferrous sulfate. Consider using lower, more frequent doses of gentler forms such as ferrous picolinate, or herbal blend liquids such as Floradix Iron Plus Herbs. I have observed children to manage these much better. Ferrous sulfate may be more constipating than these, and challenging for children with problems using any compounds that quickly give additional sulfur. Children with untreated bowel infections may tolerate iron especially poorly. Disruptive microbes in the gut may thrive with the additional iron; this may trigger a bloom of microbial organic acids that may be quite irritating. Likewise, dosing a child with iron when he is ill with a fever may not be advisable either, so check with your pediatrician. Inflammation can alter diagnostics for iron status, so if your child has a chronic inflammatory condition such as asthma, cystic fibrosis, Crohn's disease, or autism (in which more frequent inflammation from foods and bowel infections has been noted), thoughtful assessment of his capacity to absorb nutrients and for inflammatory markers may help your doctor dose an iron supplement safely and more effectively.

Iron metabolism is complicated, especially when there are chronic conditions, inflammation, or entrenched malnutrition in the picture—any of which can be true for a special-needs child. For example, a correlation has been noted between higher levels of iron in blood and poorer blood sugar control for those with diabetes. Those with autism appear to have special circumstances around iron, too. Some children with autism seem to be particularly sensitive to iron supplements. In one review of 3,000 patients with autism, about a third had too much iron in their blood. This can be so toxic that it may cause oxidative stress in the brain, meaning that nerve cells can be damaged by it. Since one theory of autism relates to damage caused by oxidative stress, the researchers wondered if iron toxicity contributes to this. Have your pediatrician do a thorough assessment of the iron status markers mentioned above, if there is any question.

Conversely, I have encountered kids with autism who *were* anemic and who have responded very well to correct supplementation with iron. This is yet another example of why *individualized nutrition care is so important for special-needs children*. There is no one-size-fits-all approach to using supplements or special diets. Some research shows that children with autism were found to have anemia more often than children with Asperger's syndrome or their neurotypical peers. This can happen to any child who has chronic loose stool, a poor food intake, or chronic problems digesting and absorbing food. Interestingly, insomnia was among the symptoms that improved in these children when iron was replenished.

Of course, pump up the iron-rich foods if you can. Certain foods enhance iron uptake (citrus, vitamin C, and acid foods such as tomato sauce; even iron cookware can help), while others block it (fiber and oxalates, as in spinach). Iron from meats occurs in a form called heme iron and this is most easily absorbed by the human gut, along with iron, in human breast milk—which has less iron than formulas, but is better absorbed. Nonheme iron is in many plant foods, such as lentils, broccoli, spinach, soy foods, quinoa, lima beans, and kidney beans.

Take a peek at copper. Elevated copper has been associated with various psychiatric diagnoses since the 1960s, when it was first noted in patients with schizophrenia. Too much copper is toxic to the brain; too little can trigger another type of anemia. In recent years, children with autism have been found to also have unusually high levels of copper in some cases, along with far too little zinc. If your child is struggling with autism, bipolar features, hyperactivity, or violent behavior, checking copper status may be fruitful. Most copper in blood (about 85–95 percent) is supposed to be carried safely in a protein called ceruloplasmin, not free and unbound as copper alone—the latter form acts as a free radical that becomes toxic. Your doctor can start by checking both ceruloplasmin level and serum copper level to determine this ratio for your child. If ceruloplasmin is too low and unbound copper is high, supplementing zinc (starting at 15 milligrams and increasing to 30 or 40 milligrams per day in some cases) can help excrete the excess copper. Your child will also need free amino acids readily available to do this, too, to form a protein called metallothionein, which will capture the copper for excretion. Use SHS North America Essential Amino Acid Mix or Kirkman Amino Support Powder for this purpose.

Include supporting cast members. If your child's CBC shows some shifts toward larger, fewer red blood cells along with questionable iron status, you will want to add vitamin B12 to your supplement plan along with iron. B12 is a safe, very low toxicity nutrient that many children with autism and ADHD appear to struggle with, in terms of its metabolic functionality in the brain. For building healthy, oxygen-toting red blood cells, you can easily give your child a boost with a sublingual B12 melting tablet or spray along with whatever iron dose your doctor suggests. You can also use a high-potency children's multivitamin that delivers the whole cast of B-group vitamins, such as ProThera VitaTab chewables, Klaire Labs VitaSpectrum Powder, or Kirkman's Children's Chewable wafers. B vitamins have exceedingly low toxicity. Too much B6 (aka pyridoxine or "P5P") can make children hyper or wakeful. If you notice agitation in your child after giving high-dose B vitamins, try another product that gives more ordinary levels. In any case, iron is a very important nutrient for learning, focus, and cognition—one that your pediatrician can help you assess and manage.

Give adequate total calories. This is the base layer for any child, a necessary foundation for functioning throughout the day. While obesity is escalating in our pediatric population, many special-needs children struggle with a poor growth pattern and under-weight. Underweight is clinically defined as being in less than the 5th percentile in weight for age, and/or less than the 10th percentile in body mass index (BMI) for age. This means your child is too thin for his height. Children who are clinically underweight have a lot more challenges than ideal weight children ("ideal body weight" has a clinical definition, too, so none of these terms are subjective). They get sick more frequently, tend to have a more challenging course of illness when they do get sick, and can have more trouble with cognition, behavior, focus, and concentration. Even if your child is overweight (above the 85th percentile in BMI for age) or obese (above the 95th percentile in BMI for age), appropriate levels of calories throughout the day are necessary for best learning.

It is common for children with special needs not to eat enough, secondary to self-limited eating patterns, nausea or anxiety before school, as a side effect of medications (especially stimulants such as methylphenidate), swallowing disorders, allergies, or oral tactile hypersensitivity. If your child has any of these issues, a check on their total daily intake is wise. I routinely find that children eat marginal diets—not because they have bad parents, but because the challenges to good eating overwhelm the child. *Special-Needs Kids Eat Right* is my step-by-step guide to walk parents through the process of improving food intakes, using special diet strategies, choosing lab tests, and more. Check that book for details on successful strategies. See the resources section of this book for a quick screen on calories, proteins, and fats needed daily in children.

If you are struggling to make a sack lunch—or any meals—that accommodate your child's food allergies or special diet needs, check out My Food My Health on the web. This is a subscription-based site that lets you enter your own diet or health concerns; it then creates customized menus, meal plans, recipes, and shopping lists around whatever foods you need to avoid. For families, this site makes accommodating a special diet much easier, in that it helps you prepare meals that everyone can enjoy at once—no more cooking separate dishes for separate kids! There are also ample helpful freebies there for everything from food-medication interactions, to free recipes organized by health condition, to food safety—and even details on antioxidant levels in foods. I often refer patients to this site. My Food My Health has generously offered a 15 percent discount off their subscription price to readers of this book. Simply input the code SNKGPF, the initials of this book, when you sign up. See the resources section for more websites that can help you plan meals around special diet needs.

If your child has obstacles eating at school because of food allergies, you should know that by law, public schools are required to accommodate him by offering children safe foods to eat at school. Children with autism following gluten-free, casein-free diets may gain access to this accommodation; you may need to produce a doctor's note justifying the accommodation. Though the law is well intended, districts vary with their capacity and willingness to comply with it. If you would like to learn what is workable in your child's cafeteria, ask to speak to your district's food and nutrition services director (did you know there was one?). Here in Boulder, where I live, we are fortunate to have an initiative under way for healthier school lunches. This has brought us options such as a fresh salad bar, organic and local source ingredients, fresh-cooked meals rather than meals that are prepackaged and reheated, occasional gluten-free options on the menu, and no more corn syrup or additives in school foods. For more information on what your school district might be able to do, visit chef Ann Cooper on the web. One of my favorite features on her site is her database of quantity recipes that are healthy, taste good to kids, and that comply with federal school lunch guidelines—so they are ready for any school kitchen to consider or implement.

When kids won't eat during the school day, I often turn to a medical food called Splash. This is a hypoallergenic liquid nutrition option for children over one year old with gastrointestinal impairment or multiple food allergies—in plain English, it's a special juice box. Not juice at all but a carefully formulated drink that can't trigger inflammation but can replenish your child. It also works well for kids with oral tactile hypersensitivity, chewing or swallowing disorders, or processing deficits so deep that they can't manage to eat in a busy environment such as a school cafeteria. Splash is an amalgam of individual nutrients that are ready to absorb and require minimal to no digestion. It is higher calorie than whole milk, and has more vitamins and minerals, too. Because it contains vitamins and minerals children need, plus macronutrients, it is a "complete food," which has a specific meaning as far as the FDA is concerned. It has a complete protein source (from free essential amino acids), an easy-to-absorb fat source (medium chain triglycerides from coconut and some sunflower and canola oils), and maltodextrin from nongenetically modified corn. In a perfect world, its carbohydrate source would be something other than maltodextrin from corn, which some kids don't tolerate well, and which many parents refuse outright owing to concerns about corn in general. But for parents willing to try it, it can work very well to sustain children during the school day, even if they don't manage to eat a bite. For many underweight children in my practice, I have used this product to replenish them when all other options have failed. For other lunch ideas for kids on special diets, visit NutritionCare.net for updates on resources for parents.

How to Increase Appetite for Adequate Total Calories

When appetites are weaker than they should be, a child struggles to eat enough food to fuel normal growth and functioning. It is not okay to shrug and say "she's just petite" if your child is actually in growth regression, a status that is quickly noted on growth history charts. Simply telling parents to feed their children more isn't useful, nor are vague assurances that "she probably gets enough food." A common strategy is to put kids on higher-calorie drinks such as Boost or Ensure, but this will backfire if the protein in those drinks is a source of inflammation. It usually is. If your child has tried a tool like that and hasn't rebounded quickly, this is a sign that this food is not being tolerated or absorbed very well. More of it isn't going to do much good—in fact, it will do more harm than good, by triggering chronic immune responses, tissue damage from inflammation, or irritable stools. Switch to the Splash elemental formula mentioned above; it may get your child going in the right direction. Here are nutrition items to check, to improve appetite, so that your child can eat enough during the day to fuel focus, attention, behavior, and learning:

Check zinc. Both insufficient and frankly deficient status for zinc (and iron) can weaken appetites. Children may begin eating more, and may even budge a self-imposed rigid repertoire of allowed foods, when these minerals are replenished. It is not at all unusual for children to be in marginal status for these minerals right here in the United States. Children can safely use 20 milligrams of zinc daily. To rule out whether more is needed for specific circumstances (like excess copper in blood or for heavy metal chelation protocols), talk to a licensed health care provider. Zinc and iron compete for absorption. If your child uses supplements for both, give them on alternating days or at opposite ends of the day. Children using more than 30 milligrams of zinc daily over the long term may drive iron status downward and trigger iron deficiency. If you routinely supplement zinc for your child, you may want your pediatrician to check iron status, especially in a child who avoids iron-rich foods such as red meat, lentils, kidney beans, fortified cereals or grains (Cream of Rice, breakfast cereals), broccoli, or bok choy.

Back to bowel flora. Another reliable way to improve appetite in children, both for quantity and for variety, is to treat bowel infections. There's no harm in using sneaky tactics to hide healthy fruits or vegetables in foods for kids, but ordinarily, a kid's appetite should be flexible enough so that parents don't need to go to such lengths. Get the best of both worlds by learning a few new recipes that use healthy vegetables or fruits, *and* improve your child's appetite and absorption by treating bowel infections. If your child self-limits his diet to fewer than eight or ten foods, odds are (in my experience) there is an entrenched bowel infection. I meet many children who have been through feeding clinics, in which the rigid eating pattern is regarded as mostly behavioral in origin. But behavioral interventions are doomed to fail when there are underlying nutrition problems left untreated. The most elusive of these may be bowel infections, since this is a new area of research that has probably not yet trickled down to your pediatrician's office. But for many years, I and many other providers have noticed how these interfere with how diets are accepted, absorbed, and eliminated in kids. Identifying and treating bowel infections is not difficult, once your provider accepts that they *do* play a role in appetite.

So, what are they? As described in Chapter 1, bowel infections are overgrowths of microbes in the gut that cause more havoc than health. The human gut harbors countless hundreds of millions of microorganisms, and we need them. They help us digest and absorb food; they produce nutrients we need; they work with our immune systems to keep invasive viruses or other bugs out. The study of how these interact with our immune systems, especially at birth, is just emerging. Children who have needed frequent antibiotics from infancy, who were born via C-section, who spent time in intensive care as newborns, and/or who have poorly tolerated their vaccinations may have altered bowel microbe profiles. New research has begun to describe how devastating this may be to our health. Antibiotics kill beneficial gut microbes; when this is done repeatedly in infancy and early childhood, research is showing that there may be an increased risk for food allergies, asthma, and other inflammatory conditions later on. Probiotics are also successful at treating infections of more serious gut pathogens such as clostridia, which can cause diarrheal illnesses in children. To restore normal bowel flora, here are a few options:

- Use diversified strains of probiotic supplements rather than a single strain or two per supplement. Look for eight or more strains of beneficial microbes in one product.

- Use high-potency probiotics. Look for a minimum of 8–10 billion "colony forming units" (CFUs) per dose.

- Chewable probiotic tablets may not be potent enough to do much good. They often have fillers and sweeteners that do *no* good. For a faster, therapeutically relevant impact, use powdered probiotic in high potencies. Stir into soft foods or drinks, dust into sandwich spreads, or mix in warm (not hot) foods.

- Yogurt contains beneficial flora, but just eating yogurt each day probably won't change a child's rigid appetite—

especially if it's that overly sweet, artificially colored, drinkable stuff, which has more sugar than anything else in it. More aggressive measures are usually needed.

- Fermented foods such as sauerkraut, tempeh, miso, and kimchi are good helpers because they contain natural probiotics, too. If your child is adventurous and willing to eat those foods regularly, wonderful! These are low-calorie foods, so keep this in mind as you endeavor to give your child enough total calories daily. These foods are likely to interfere with, but not eradicate, bowel infections from microbes such as clostridia, klebsiella, or candida. Your child may still need treatment for these even if he eats fermented foods.

- Children with many rounds of antibiotics in their histories probably need even higher-potency products. Consider using 12–25 billion CFUs per dose in these cases.

- Consider adding an herbal antimicrobial agent to kill disruptive strains of bacteria and yeasts (candida, rhodotorula) that flourish when antibiotics are repeatedly given. Do not give these herbs and any probiotics at the same time; administer each at opposite ends of the day, to give the probiotics the best opportunity to colonize the gut.

- Herbal antimicrobials and antifungals (that is, yeast killing) are easy to give to young children. Many compounds are available in drops for this age group. Examples of these include Biocidin drops, uva ursi drops (do not use longer than one week), olive leaf extract, cranberry extract, or grapefruit seed extract drops (very pungent and best in tart drinks or water). Herbal blends for this purpose are sold as drops, too, from companies such as HerbPharm, WishGarden Herbs, or Herbs for Kids.

- Some products incorporate curcumin for its potent antimicrobial activity. Curcumin was found to be more effective than fluconazole (which you may know as Diflucan, commonly prescribed for yeast infections) against several candida species in at least one clinical trial. To use curcumin in children, work with an experienced provider. A promising curcumin product called Enhansa may be useful in cases that have been unresponsive even to prescription antifungals such as Diflucan or Nystatin, or where unwanted bacterial and viral infections persist in the child's gut.

Your child's food intake should be hearty enough to support expected growth, to allow relatively even energy levels throughout the day (rather than spikes of busy hyperactivity followed by tantrums or crashes), and to give sound sleep. If improvements just aren't forthcoming with the measures given above, then it may be time to ask your pediatrician to consider using medication to treat an intestinal fungal infection—especially if

- Appetite is so rigid or weak that growth impairment has set in. Growth impairment means your child has dropped fifteen percentage points on her growth chart in the past year or less.

- Growth failure has not resolved with other measures. Growth failure means your child has stopped gaining in height or weight for six months, or that your child has fallen from a higher percentile to the 5th percentile or lower on the growth chart.

- Stool incontinence or constipation has not resolved with other measures.

- Naturopathic efforts (probiotics, herbs) have failed to resolve these problems.

- Your child's weak and picky appetite is taking you and school staff hours to overcome on a daily basis, because you have to cajole your child into eating.

Using a medication for a fungal infection, when the right one is chosen and used at the right dosage and duration, can abruptly resolve all of these problems—I have witnessed it time and again. Your pediatrician can review for you what medication is safest to try, if your child is on other medications at the same time. Some cannot be mixed with antifungal drugs such as fluconazole. If your child has persisting problems with appetite and stooling even after a course of antifungal medication, this likely means that the infection is not entirely gone, or that other microbes have now come to the fore and need treatment. Revisit this with a stool microbiology culture from a functional medicine lab that identifies individual strains for beneficial bacteria, for fungal species, and for disruptive bacteria. This can give your provider the clearest information on what to do next.

This may sound far-fetched, but some research is now catching up with years of anecdotal accounts from parents about intestinal fungal infections in kids with ADHD, autism, or Asperger's syndrome. The more candida present on their stool cultures, the worse features are for behavior or autism, according to a few initial studies. Treating the candida overgrowth has triggered dramatic behavioral improvements for many of these children. If you are at your wit's end with a child who has barely manageable mood swings, rage reactions, or hyperactivity and inattention, see if your MD provider will allow a trial with an antifungal medication—especially if your child's history includes frequent antibiotics, C-section birth, or long-term use of reflux medication. The long-term impact of never developing normal bowel flora, as would be true for a child with that history, is barely studied. But it may well include effects on learning and behavior later on. Antifungal medications have an excellent safety record. If it will do no harm, and you have failed with psychiatric medication options, then your doctor may be willing to give it a try for you.

The same has been seen for correcting clostridia infections in children with autism. As with yeast, the wrong populations of bacteria in the gut can be very disruptive. This was stunningly illustrated in research using antibiotic treatment in children with autism. The antibiotic permitted abrupt improvement in autism features, in a landmark case series published several years ago (benefits ceased when the antibiotic was withdrawn). More recent research illustrates that a fatty acid called proprionic acid can abruptly trigger autism behaviors in normal rats, who resume their normal state once the proprionic acid is metabolized. Compelling work by a group in Canada under Derrick MacFabe, MD, shows rats going from ordinary to anxious, antisocial, and engaging in repetitive behaviors immediately after direct exposure of proprionic acid to their brains. Proprionic acid is a short chain fatty acid made by clostridia bacteria, a common resident of the human gut. Several species of clostridia bacteria may exist in the intestine, and the immune system normally keeps these in check by permitting healthy microbes to grow there instead. Emerging research implies that in autism, this balance is not maintained; some speculate that disruption of immune signaling at the gut is part of the puzzle. The result may be that proprionic acid, which can cross the blood-brain barrier as easily as alcohol, is absorbed from overgrowth of clostridia species in the gut; this in turn may cause antisocial behavior, obsessive-compulsive or repetitive behaviors, or some of the odd motor tics seen in autism. Proprionic acid in high or repeat doses has also been shown to be a trigger for seizures.

What does this mean for your child with extreme anxiety, tics, obsessive-compulsive disorder, intractable seizure disorder, or antisocial behaviors? It suggests that a thoughtful review of bowel flora is in order. Different tools can assess this, all of which have their imperfections and pitfalls. Most gastroenterologists to date are not familiar with this approach, so you may need to approach a functional medicine doctor with experience in pediatrics, or a naturopath. Usually when a child shows dramatic forward progress with it, doctors get on board and become more curious to investigate the literature. Work with a provider who has a track record in treating what is often called gut dysbiosis, to see if treatments to keep clostridia under control are warranted.

Remove inflammatory foods. For children with rigid or weak appetites, the next nutrition checkpoint after bowel infections is to identify and remove foods that trigger inflammation. The conventional wisdom in pediatrics is to let underweight kids eat unrestricted diets, and to add products such as Boost, Carnation Instant Breakfast, Ensure, or Peptamen Junior to pack in calories. This is based on an assumption that limiting their choices will limit calorie intakes. It may seem counterintuitive, but kids can and do eat *more* when diets exclude foods that bother them (and dairy protein, which is in all those products I just mentioned, is often one of the problems). While bowel infections tend to make kids' appetites rigid for just a few foods, inflammation from foods tends to make kids' appetites weak; children can have either or both of these problems at once. These are kids who just don't eat enough, who need a lot of coaxing or distractions to get the food in, who can't sit through a meal, who graze lightly and rarely eat meals, or who don't develop typically around feeding themselves. Parents often come in having received medical advice *not* to restrict a child's diet at all, in order to uncork the variety they can try to eat. But this will usually backfire when the child continues eating inflammatory foods—most likely because inflammatory foods trigger insidious GI symptoms that your child may not recognize or communicate very well. Stomachaches, reflux, irritable bowels, and headaches are common features of active IgG food antibody reactions. Even highly verbal, bright, and functional children will be confused about expressing these symptoms if they have no memory of not ever having them in the first place, and this can be true for children who have never been assessed for inflammation from foods.

How do you identify inflammatory foods? Even though findings have been published for more than ten years on this subject, most doctors still do not acknowledge anything other than classic IgE-mediated allergy as relevant for children. This means that your child might only be screened with a skin prick RAST test, or a blood RAST test. Certainly, when inflammation from foods is noted on that test, some new diet strategies are in order. But

RAST tests are frequently entirely negative, while signs for inflammation are active: irritable or loose stool pattern, bloating, stomachaches, eczema that comes and goes, mood or sensory irritability, asthma, rhinitis, frequent upper respiratory or ear infections. If any of those things are a regular part of your child's life, or particularly if you are needing medications to manage them on a frequent basis, then your child probably has some undetected inflammation from foods. All these symptoms can improve if you identify those foods and correctly replace them.

The test I rely on for that piece is an ELISA IgG food antibody panel, discussed in Chapter 3. Providers knowledgeable with this piece will use a lab that specializes in this test, which lets them assess reactivity to dozens of foods with a very small sample of blood. Some labs offer ELISA analysis that uses only five drops of blood, which means you can avoid traditional venipuncture for your child (as long as you are comfortable using a lancet in your child's toe or fingertip). See the resources section for information on labs that do this test. It will not be informative in children younger than eighteen to twenty months old, whose immature immune systems may show false positives on the panel. In this age group, elimination diets are more reliable for identifying problem foods.

I have heard opposition to this test over the years, mostly from providers who have not used it in practice, or who may not have stayed abreast of the research on it. I have also had hundreds of conversations with parents about this. Yes, there is published peer review on this test. Having used it for a decade, I can attest that it has reliably guided me on prioritizing foods in a child's diet. One objection I can agree with: Results of an ELISA panel should not become a mandate to remove all reactive foods that pop up.

It becomes too difficult to meet the nutritional needs of children when you eliminate four or more major protein sources. If your child has inflammation or allergy from more than four foods, professional guidance is helpful, so you can confidently rebuild your child's food choices in the healthiest way. Which foods should be prioritized for removal and how to replenish those is best done on an individualized basis. Children avoiding this many foods may need an amino acid protein source, a hydrolyzed source, or an augmented rice source. There are many options, and it's best to get professional guidance when using this test.

Make sure protein sources are well tolerated. As described above, inflammation from food proteins can trigger irritability, worsen sensory processing disorders, and worsen impulsivity. Feeding a child a chronically inflammatory diet worsens distractibility, attention, and focus, too. The most commonly problematic proteins in this scenario are casein and dairy proteins, gluten, and soy. Gluten sensitivity in particular may trigger neurological effects such as anxiety, tremors, involuntary eye movements, or cognitive deficits. While some contend that there is no link between gluten and these symptoms, research has emerged over the last decade that describes a cross-reactivity between gliadin antibodies and brain tissue. Gliadin is a portion of gluten, which is the protein in wheat (and some other grains). A blood test can check for antigliadin antibodies; if they are present, this means that wheat triggers inflammation in that individual. If your immune system makes antibodies to gliadin, this is an aberrant inflammatory response that shouldn't be happening. In itself, it may injure gut mucosa or skin, as well as raise risk for certain cancers. If that weren't bad enough, the cross-reactivity findings mean these antibodies, intended for gliadin, attack brain tissue in an autoimmune mix-up.

Some postulate that this is why children with autism and ADHD may improve on gluten-free diets.*

Children who have either classic allergy reactions (e.g., positive IgE or RAST tests) or food sensitivity reactions (positive IgG or ELISA findings) can improve when inflammation is controlled, minimized, or eradicated. Gluten sensitivity is ruled out with a gliadin antibody blood test, not a blood test for celiac disease, which only looks at antibodies to enzymes and proteins that appear once you have celiac disease. Gluten sensitivity may be active even in persons without celiac disease. If you are wondering whether your child has inflammation from gluten, ask your doctor for an antigliadin IgG antibody test, not a celiac test.

What if it's positive? Trial a gluten-free diet. Even if it's only marginally positive, but your child has active signs for inflammation, trial a gluten-free diet for four months. Keep a dispassionate record of things such as the number of tantrums, appetite, growth (clothes fitting?), sensory meltdowns or issues, notes from school about good or bad days, stooling issues, or stomach complaints. Unless you've found that your child actually has celiac disease, in which a gluten-free diet often triggers fast relief, changes may occur with subtlety and be hard to notice otherwise. Your child does not need to be aware of the record keeping, unless it is motivating and helpful to self-esteem. If it isn't, quietly keep your own notes, and decide after a fair gluten-free trial what works best—gluten or no gluten.

* If your child did not improve on a gluten-free diet, see *Special-Needs Kids Eat Right* for an explanation of why this can fail, and strategies to make this approach work.

Make sure protein is not malabsorbed as opiate-like peptides. Food-sourced protein fragments, or "peptides," can mimic the action of opiates in the brain. They are formed when wheat (gluten), dairy (casein), and soy proteins are not completely broken down, and these peptides are now famously implicated in the symptoms of autism. When these are active, a child will lag in progress for expressive language, language praxis,* reciprocal play, expression of empathy, social referencing, and self-modulation. He may develop obsessive interests or habits. Tasks such as making even simple transitions or following instructions with more than a couple steps will be quite hard in the context of active diet-source opiates. The child may have dilated pupils especially after eating wheat, dairy, or soy foods; a diet fiercely self-limited to wheat, dairy, or soy foods; stormy tantrums if denied foods he prefers; firm or constipated stools; mood changes relative to eating; and sometimes a disrupted sleep pattern. Parents also often note a feature of being oddly impervious to pain in kids with active dietary opiate chemistry. All of these can interfere with learning, reasonable compliance in a child, and development.

A simple urine polypeptide test can rule out if these opiates are active. See the resources section for information on this test. Even when the urine test falls in range, if a child has active signs and symptoms for opiate-like chemistry, a gluten-free, casein-free (GFCF) diet may work, as long as other nutrition problems are corrected, too. Soy is usually avoided, or at least dramatically minimized, on this diet as well. Using a complete essential free

---

* Language praxis is the smooth organization of receptive and expressive language, which permits us to hear, interpret, and respond typically in conversation.

amino acid protein source, at least 8–10 grams per day, for children on GFCF diets seems to trigger additional progress cognitively and behaviorally, and sleep patterns improve. Though this area needs more study for children with autism, ADHD, or learning and mood issues, using free essential amino acids in children with GI impairment has been safely done for many years already. I suspect that more data will show that children with autism spectrum disorders, ADHD, or learning and mood issues may not typically extract amino acids from the protein in their diets, and that this leaves them bereft of precursor molecules needed for attention, focus, learning, memory, and self-modulation. In the meantime, it is easy and safe to deliver these amino acid precursors needed for brain balance simply by adding them to foods or using them in specialized formulas. For example, Kirkman Labs sells a product called Amino Support Powder, which offers a few grams of an essential amino acid blend that can be mixed into juices or soft foods. Try this in the morning with breakfast to see if your child's demeanor, affect, or focus might respond. Two teaspoons is a very reasonable amount to start; this delivers about the same amount of protein as a cup of milk, but in a form that is ready to absorb and requires no digestion to break it down.

If diet-sourced opiates are a problem, it does not work very well to avoid only one of the opiate-forming proteins of gluten, casein, and soy. Usually, all must be withdrawn; otherwise progress will be lackluster or intermittent. Tips on doing this safely and effectively can be found in *Special-Needs Kids Eat Right*. Some success is reported with using certain digestive enzymes instead of dietary restriction, or with a partial restriction. If you choose this route, you will need an enzyme called dipeptidyl-peptidase IV. This is highly specific for breaking up peptides from gluten, casein, and soy, and is incorporated into products from Kirkman Labs, Houston Enzymes, or Klaire Labs. Ordinary proteases may not be effective.

Once opiate chemistry is corrected, you can expect improved communication, both receptive and expressive, in your child; fewer tantrums; some flexibility for food choices; better emotional self-regulation; improved sleep; more comfortable bowel habits; and more attentiveness and participation at school. If these improvements don't ensue, your child may need other nutrition supports that have been overlooked. Visit NutritionCare.net for more information, support, or to schedule a consult, or pick up a copy of *Special-Needs Kids Eat Right* for step-by-step planning for successfully using a GFCF diet protocol.

Make sure magnesium is adequate. Magnesium is a key mineral for smooth nerve impulse transmission, and it is needed for some three hundred metabolic functions in cells. Foods that deliver magnesium include black beans, avocado, figs, lima beans, white beans, cornmeal, spinach, almonds, pine nuts, tofu, and cashews. Does your kid eat those foods every day? If the answer is yes, fantastic—but I often find that kids have marginal magnesium intakes, and positive clinical signs for marginal magnesium status, when I review their food diaries. When they are also presenting with hyperactivity, anxiety, irritability, insomnia, learning problems, or motor control issues, I don't need a blood test to tell me they probably need magnesium. The keynote of marginal magnesium in school-age children is often hyperactivity with inattention. This is a nutrient that has also been depleted from our soils from decades of farming techniques that use elemental fertilizers over organic, soil-building methods. So the cashews available in 1965 may have had more magnesium than the ones you bought yesterday at the supermarket, unless you sprang for the organic ones. Some nutrients, including magnesium, can shift significantly in foods, relative to how those foods were cultivated. Buying organic is one way to get a bit more magnesium into your body.

Besides offering organic sources of magnesium-rich foods to kids, using Epsom salts nightly in a ten- or fifteen-minute bath (1 cup for school-age children, ½ cup for toddlers) is a sure way to deliver it into tissues. If your child is not yet successfully accepting some of the foods above daily, supplementation can get you over the hump also. Oral magnesium supplements are used as ingredients in laxatives, so don't combine these with laxatives you already use or add high doses of magnesium without professional guidance. Excessive magnesium can cause diarrhea, heart palpitations, muscle tremors, headaches, or blood sugar fluctuations. Magnesium is stored to some extent in bone; excessive use of magnesium over time can leave too much in bone, thus making bones too soft. It can also interact with some drugs, including antibiotics. Talk to your pharmacist or doctor if your child is on a medication before adding magnesium, especially if your child must use laxatives, some of which contain magnesium. Do not exceed 300 milligrams of magnesium daily for a child without professional supervision. When it is correctly replenished, your child should show more calm and focus, and may be able to sleep better, too. Magnesium alone is not going to fix all the problems any child has, but lacking it will certainly interfere with progress.

Many products combine magnesium with other supplements in powders or liquids, especially calcium. This can work well at bedtime for children who have trouble sleeping. If constipation is on your child's fix-it list, and you are not using a laxative, try a product such as BlueBonnet Liquid Calcium and Magnesium, which has magnesium citrate in it. This is more laxative than most other forms of magnesium. If your child has diarrhea or loose stools often but still needs magnesium supplemented, use Epsom salts in the tub, or try a product such as Ionic Fizz, which provides elemental forms of magnesium that are quick to absorb and less likely to trigger diarrhea.

Maximize the benefits of omega-3 oils. We have all heard plenty about these oils. You should know that they have shown impressive results in clinical trials for mood disorders, for reducing inflammation, for interrupting proliferation of tumor cells, and for attention and focus. But which ones do you use for a child, and how much? Using something generically labeled "fish oil" or "omega-3" will probably do little good. A school-age child who is struggling with focus and attention can be given at least 400 milligrams of DHA (docosahexaenoic acid) per day, and more is appropriate if this dose doesn't trigger a benefit. Up to 800 or 1000 milligrams per day may be beneficial for some children; much higher doses (more than 10 grams) have been safely consumed by humans in clinical trials, and as a matter of habit, by certain populations that eat a lot of fish. This is the omega-3 fatty acid that has shown promise for its impact on dyslexia, focus, and attention. ADHD is associated with low levels of DHA, as are aggression and hostility. For children with mood concerns, bipolar features, depression, or who need to bracket mood swings, the omega-3 oil to focus on is EPA (eicosapentanoic acid), and the amount to start with is 800 milligrams per day for small children. Older children may need more, say 1–3 grams per day. In one trial with bipolar adult subjects, 9 grams of EPA were given daily with no ill effects, but with startling benefits affecting their mood disorder.

Both oils are deliverable via a variety of products, which vary for quality. Fish oil supplements are one class of products on which you will not want to cut corners. Fish concentrate toxins from the ocean in their livers and fatty tissues. Some companies use costlier production and quality control methods to remove these toxins, such as Nordic Naturals. See the resources section for options on giving fish oils to children. If you've been using supplemental oils for a while and have not seen progress, remember that these oils may take weeks or months to be incorporated into nerve and brain cell membranes, where they are most beneficial. You can also request a blood test that checks what fatty acids may be most needed for your child—see the resources section for more info. These oils, just like a medication, are needed daily on a consistent basis to have a therapeutic effect. Dabbling with them won't do much good. Just as you would with a medication, commit to it and try it faithfully for at least six weeks before stopping. One seven-year-old child I worked with began using 800 milligrams of EPA daily; after just three weeks, his daily severe tantrums and meltdowns had dropped to about a third of what they were before. At our next follow-up, things had deteriorated. Going back over our care plan, I asked the mom if the EPA was still being used and at what dose. She had cut the dose in half, not realizing that it mattered. It did!

Meanwhile, make sure your child's diet has plenty of other healthy oils and fats, which generally should supply about a third of your child's total calories. Coconut milk and coconut kefir or yogurt are stellar options (though void of protein, they do provide good fats). Note that I am not suggesting hydrogenated or processed coconut oil products, but fresh whole coconut milk or yogurt. Incorporate coconut milk into smoothies, baked goods, or curries, especially if your child can't tolerate cow's milk. You can also cook with coconut oil if your recipe works with this strong flavor. Allow ghee if butter must be removed; add olive oil to dips such as hummus or bean dips; try guacamole for dipping and offer soft, ripe avocado slices in sandwiches where your child may have expected a slice of cheese, if that is an allergen. Rotate allowable nut butters or snack on nuts. Only children who are managing obesity might consider a restricted fat intake, and even then, my first scrutiny would be placed on their total calorie and carbohydrate intakes—since eating a lot of sugary carbs will elevate blood lipids, cholesterol, and weight.

Doing just the things listed so far may make a good dent in your child's trouble with focus, mood, and attention, because you have given a platform for your child to stand on with adequate total food intake, better absorption in the gut, less inflammation from foods, and a few key learning nutrients. Once you have covered those bases, if your child needs more help, you can move on to specific neurotransmitter supports.

Targeting Brain Balance with Nutrition Tools

There may be no greater need in our pediatric population today than this. As the numbers of children with autism, ADHD, learning problems, and mood disorders climb, tools that can help balance brain chemistry are in more demand than ever before for youngsters. Pharmaceuticals for this job have been pushed to the fore for over a decade. In spite of some tragic outcomes with psychotropic medications, as well as lackluster results for some children, MD providers have little to draw upon to make other recommendations. While it's true that comparatively little published research is available on nutrients for psychiatric diagnoses, there is not *none*; in fact, there is quite a bit of it. But given biases in medical journals for reviewing pharmaceutical treatments over nonpharm treatments, and given the colossal resources of the pharmaceutical industry for marketing and underwriting research, it is an uphill battle to inform doctors on nondrug strategies. The entire pharmaceutical industry is worth some $300 billion in the United States alone each year, while the entire supplement industry here barely registers less than 1 percent of that amount, for its total sales on an annual basis.

We can expand the toolbox for these conditions in children by adding nutrition-focused options. Some of them are presented here, while others are beyond the scope of this book, and beyond my scope in practice. For resources that surpass what I can describe here, visit "Commentary on Nutritional Treatment of Mental Disorders," at AlternativeMentalHealth.com. A series of articles there by William Walsh, PhD, outline numerous treatable nutritional deficits and aberrations seen in persons with psychoses as severe as paranoid schizophrenia, as well as autism, bipolar disorder, and ADHD. A scientist at the Pfeiffer Treatment Center in Illinois, Dr. Walsh describes the complex challenges in correctly assessing and treating these nutritional biochemistry imbalances, which are consistently seen in persons with psychiatric disorders. This area of practice is emerging under the "Integrative Psychiatry" moniker. It finds that—as I have found to be true for children with autism—there is no one nutritional protocol that works for all persons with a particular psychiatric diagnosis. While there may be general trends within each diagnosis (for example, most children with autism whom I work with benefit from gluten avoidance and are zinc depleted), individualized assessment and care plans are necessary for integrative psychiatry to work. It takes more commitment than leaving your pediatrician's office with a prescription for Adderall. By example, some children with obsessive-compulsive disorder may need supplements that replenish methylation pathways; others may worsen with this strategy, and a skilled practitioner in integrative psychiatry can individually assess and treat a child for this piece.

One of the most effective tools in my nutrition box is the simplest when it comes to improving attention, language effort, and appropriate social functioning: Add amino acids that we all need for certain brain states. When children have digestive problems, as described earlier in this chapter and in greater detail in *Special-Needs Kids Eat Right*, they may not send amino acids to the brain that they need for learning, focus, attention, mood, sleeping, calming, or whatever. Perhaps these amino acid precursors are not well absorbed in the first place, or perhaps dietary opiates or organic acids from bowel infections are interfering with brain chemistry. Myriad other interferences may exist. In any case, adding essential amino acid blends, or giving individual amino acids in a bolus dose (a larger single dose than might normally come from a meal), can replenish and feed pathways that make our own neurotransmitters. A short list of amino tools to consider follows some need-to-know items for parents of children who have serious learning, attention, or mood concerns.

Get professional support. Children struggling with stress, depression, anxiety, or conduct disorders should be evaluated and supported by a knowledgeable pediatric psychiatrist (MD) or psychologist (PhD) provider. Even young children can have obsessive-compulsive tendencies, mood swings that raise the specter of bipolar disorder, hyperactivity so pronounced that teachers refuse to work with the child, or anxiety and depression so entrenched that school is out of the question. Start with a conversation with your pediatrician, and ask for a referral to an experienced specialist. Your child may need other therapies besides nutrition tools that support learning, cognition, and behavior, including play or talk therapies, pharmaceuticals, or more. Get more than one professional opinion if possible. It's easy to forget that children with special needs can be more stressed by the usual demands of school and activities; they may simply need a lot more downtime than you might expect. Even for typical peers, the pressures placed on children for performance are higher than ever. Get professional guidance on when it's appropriate to implement a medication or nutrition support, and when it's best to let your child just process the many demands in his life with some unscheduled, unstructured playtime.

Protect your child's right to FAPE. FAPE is "free and appropriate education," which all children are entitled to in the United States, regardless of their disability status, under the mandate of the Individuals with Disabilities in Education Act. Many children in my practice are so affected by psychiatric issues that they either can't attend school because it's overwhelming or they lose their school placements because administrators and teachers are unsupportive to the point of seeking a way to remove the child, against the family's wishes. This is contentious, traumatic territory for children and families—and unfortunately, more common than you might think. Once a school district decides they no longer want to accommodate a child in a regular classroom, teachers and administrators may work to see that goal through, whether it's legal or illegal, ethical or unethical, or in the child's best interest or not. Much of this is driven by budget crises in schools today—it's simply too costly to add staff or resources for children who need extra help. Meanwhile, parents of neurotypical children complain about disruptive learners in the classroom, and may pressure staff to have them removed, not knowing that this is a civil rights violation.

In other instances I have encountered with families, children who perform poorly on state standards tests are driven out of a school, if the school is desperate to maintain high scores that earn them funding. (Under the No Child Left Behind legislation, schools with low scores are "punished" by losing funding.) If you are being told your child must leave his placement in a public school, don't confide in school staff or ask them for advice. Anything you say or put in writing can be used against your child at this point. Seek independent legal advice posthaste. It is also illegal for school staff to tell you that your child must be medicated in order to attend school.

If you suspect that your child's rights to education access are being violated, investigate with reputable sources beyond your school team. School staff may be too mired in other motivations and needs to advocate for your child anymore. The right to free and appropriate education is explicitly protected by federal law, no matter what your child's disability is. See the resources section for a list of organizations that provide counsel and information on the rights of children with special needs in public schools. Private schools are generally free to admit or exclude children at their discretion, but federal law protects access to education in the public school system for all learners.

Happily, I have helped children preserve school placements

through nutrition measures. Some of these children were using psychiatric medication already; some had tried medication and failed with it; some had not tried any yet at all. Others eliminated medications because nutrition tools were more successful, while some found medications more effective when used with nutrition tools and kept both. The point is to surround your family with a supportive, knowledgeable team of professionals who help your child feel and function better.

The Right Nutrition Can Support Neurotransmitters for Learning and Focus

Nutrition tools such as amino acids have the advantage of being very safe, having no side effects, and working fast. Usually a clear benefit is detectable on the first day, sometimes within minutes; at the longest, a few days may be needed to really establish if you are seeing a benefit. If there is a negative response or no response, aminos leave the body rapidly. There is no need to build up an effective dose as is often true when using psychotropic medications in children. When adding amino acids, remember to also supply a high-potency multivitamin and mineral supplement for your child, to cover bases on needed cofactors that create neurotransmitters out of amino acids—especially for B vitamins. Your child will also need aminos delivered in the context of adequate total calories from carbohydrates and fats, in order to assure that protein and amino acids are not wasted for meeting energy and growth needs.

Start simple. A simple check of whether or not your child's neurotransmitter chemistry is bereft of amino acids it may need is to give an essential amino acid blend in the morning, with a mostly carb breakfast—say waffles, bagel, hot rice or oat cereal, or toast. Mix about 5 grams (1 teaspoon) of a blend of essential free amino acids into a smoothie, shake, applesauce, or warm (not hot) rice cereal. I usually use SHS North America Essential Amino Acid Mix for this purpose, which is a medical-grade blend of only the amino acids humans can't make in their own chemistry—hence the term "essential," meaning they are essential to life. This product was created for use in modular tube feedings, that is, in hospital settings where children are tube fed and must have a protein source that is highly absorbable and cannot trigger inflammation. See the resources section for information on this and other amino acid blends to try (I've even requested a custom formulation for my practice, since finding the right one can be hard). Using more than 2 teaspoons (10 grams) of free amino acids at once may be too agitating for some children, especially to start, and especially in formulations that include tyrosine. Tyrosine is considered "conditionally essential" in that some circumstances make it hard for us to make enough of it. It has a stimulatory effect that you can learn more about later in this chapter.

Especially for the first few tries with this tool, it's best not to mix it with milk or eat the aminos with other high-protein foods. This is because the milk or food protein's amino acids will compete for absorption with the supplemented free amino acids for entry into the brain. Likewise, don't mix free amino acids with protein powders from soy, dairy, whey, casein, egg, or rice. The idea is to preferentially push certain neurotransmitter pathways with a ready supply of the amino acids that the brain needs to build them. By giving the supplemental amino acids with some carbohydrate calories and not food protein, you will enhance their uptake into the brain and eliminate competition; this can give you a clearer picture of your child's response.

In 1999, I first used this approach in children with autism, by placing them on a free amino acid formula made for gastrointestinal impairment and food allergy. These children did better with their special diet interventions than children with autism on special diets who did not use a free amino acid protein source, even when both groups got adequate calories and total protein from food sources. This implies that the availability of those amino acids for brain chemistry is part of the puzzle for children with autism; the same may apply for those with ADHD or other learning challenges, though to a different degree. The FDA has recently approved a clinical trial that incorporates this approach from another angle: An enzyme that accelerates protein digestion is being tested in kids with autism based on the hypothesis that they do not normally liberate amino acids from foods, and thus have deficits in neurotransmitters. It will be interesting to see how this goes. Meanwhile, simply feeding the amino acids orally can be effective, too—though this is still being studied. Anecdotally, parents have shared that their children have become more aware, more verbal, and more engaged when given free amino acids.

Amino acids are simply protein components that are normally extracted from food; the difference with using an amino acid blend as described here is that you are providing the components in a ready-to-absorb state that requires no digestion, for quick entry into the brain. A dose of 8–10 grams is ordinary, and no more than would be in 8–10 ounces of milk as intact protein. Still, if your child has a seizure disorder, it's best to check with your provider first. The resources section lists other vendors that sell free amino acids, which should not be confused with products such as soy or rice protein powders.

Some providers prescribe custom compounded blends of amino acids, based on analysis of urine samples that check neurotransmitter metabolites. I have not yet observed this to be as successful as I would have hoped. It is hard to discern through urine samples exactly what is going on in nerve synapses in the brain. Blood levels of neurotransmitters don't necessarily reflect brain levels either. These panels also can't inform completely on other nutrients besides aminos that are needed for brain balance, and they say nothing at all about total food intakes, which are critical for normal mood, sleep, energy level, and affect in children. Just as is done with psychiatric medications, it can work well to use history, signs, and symptoms to choose an amino acid supplement rather than costly lab studies. For children, history should include a review of total intakes for calories, proteins, fats, and carbs, too.

Attention and focus. If an essential amino blend did nothing for your child, try tyrosine, the go-to amino acid for attention and focus. Tyrosine is a precursor for dopamine; dopamine is the neurotransmitter responsible for a sense of motivation, and for telling our brains to pay attention. It is active when we experience pleasure, or when we learn and remember stuff effectively. Normal dopamine chemistry is critical for problem solving. Too little of it in certain areas of the brain is thought to create attention deficit disorder, social anxiety, and social withdrawal; way too little of it may trigger movement disorders. Parkinson's disease is a condition in which far too little dopamine is present. Dopamine excess can produce symptoms of schizophrenia or mania, addictive behavior, or obsessive-compulsive behaviors. Dopamine is the neurotransmitter upstream of epinephrine and norepinephrine in our chemistry, so if it is imbalanced, these chemicals will be, too. Though some providers use urine tests to assess neurotransmitters, these are indirect, imperfect measures that can't emphatically describe something like dopamine or serotonin levels in the brain. To round out your baseline information on which neurotransmitters need correcting for your child, work with a knowledgeable mental health professional who can help you ascertain this, based on signs, symptoms, and behaviors.

Children and teens who are typically unable to focus or pay attention, and who are being considered for a stimulant medication, are candidates for tyrosine supplementation. You can also consider this if your child has been unsuccessful with methylphenidate drugs because of side effects such as headaches, irritability, crashing and fierce crabbiness late in the day when their stimulant medication wears off, or if a stimulant medication has diminished appetite so much that your child is underweight (body mass index below the 10th percentile) or growth has regressed. Children who are already struggling to maintain a normal growth pattern are also excellent candidates for pharm-free approaches to inattention, since a side effect of stimulant medications for some is depressed appetite and weight loss. You can also try tyrosine before using a medication to see if it is successful enough in itself. An individual who needs tyrosine may have these signs and symptoms:

- Is slow and sluggish to get going in the morning

- Has pronounced inattention at school; can't stay organized

- Suffers from a low mood, low energy, low affect

- Avoids exercise and physical activity; is sedentary

- Feels chronically stressed and overwhelmed by the demands of school

- Is drained by a stressful event such as moving, major changes in family life, switching schools, chronic bullying, or worrying about grades

- Is usually unable to finish work at school; papers are half done

- Is unable to write at grade level; can't fill a page or complete a paragraph, or can't take notes in class

- Is drawn to stimulants such as alcohol, coffee, tea, cigarettes, and sugary foods[*]

If school staff and your provider team truly feel it is appropriate to intervene for focus and attention in very young children at all, tyrosine is a safe and easy-to-use option. Preschool children are given more stimulant prescriptions than any other psychotropic medication. The long-term effects of stimulants on the developing brain are not well studied, and many parents are hesitant to begin with these, when wondering how to help a child focus typically. In practice, I usually find that when young children (under five years or so) are behaving in such an unwieldy fashion as to warrant a visit to the psychologist, nutrition measures can be employed to improve behavior at home and at school. The

---

[*] While most kids like sweets, a refusal to eat other healthier foods as well, with extreme rigidity for starchy foods and sweets, is not normal.

usual suspects in that regard are treating bowel infections, avoiding inflammatory foods, reducing sugary intakes, improving protein intakes, correctly supplementing omega-3 fatty acids, and replenishing minerals (especially zinc, magnesium, selenium, and chromium). I may then try the essential amino acid blend in the morning for these youngsters, if more is needed. Those tools usually do the trick, and we find that it isn't necessary to add individual amino acids.

For kids hitting fifth grade and up, those tricks work well, too. But school demands dramatically shift by that age. Kids are expected to produce a lot more paperwork, to sit and focus more, and have fewer chances to move around. By middle school, things get even harder. Kids may be changing classes and teachers several times a day; they have to keep all their own assignments organized; the rules of what is socially expected change virtually overnight; recess is now only a memory, so free playtime is gone. Extra help in concentrating and focusing is a welcome relief for many kids, and tyrosine can safely do this in many cases.

Tyrosine is a naturally occurring, essential amino acid* that the brain needs to make dopamine, which is the neurotransmitter responsible for paying attention. As is true for supplementing any amino acid, don't add it if your child is on a psychotropic medication without checking with your doctor first. It is readily available in capsules (usually 500 milligrams) or loose powder. For smaller children (under 60 pounds), starting with 100 milligrams of loose

---

* Tyrosine is considered "conditionally essential" for infants and children, depending on growth rates, food intakes, and status for digesting and absorbing protein.

powder in soft food such as applesauce is perhaps overly cautious, but reasonable, since we all vary with regard to status of neurotransmitter chemistry. This is a tiny dose—½ cup of chopped turkey meat has eight times more tyrosine in it. This will be a very small amount of powder, less than ⅛ teaspoon. You can also spread this on your child's morning toast with butter or jam, in hot cereal, or in thick juice or a smoothie. Tyrosine powder does not have any particularly objectionable taste. It will lighten the color of whatever food or drink it goes in, so if your child has sharp radar for changes in the appearance or texture of food, prepare him accordingly if that works best. Older children (above 80 pounds) may start with 250 milligrams, and use capsules if this is easier. "Start low and go slow" is the adage to apply for using any amino acid supplement. You can increase the dose either a day at a time or hourly, to discern what is effective for your child. Go up in small increments (by 100 milligrams) for smaller children, and larger increments (by 250 or 500 milligrams) for older children and teens. If your child has too much tyrosine, he will seem agitated in a way that you might feel with too much caffeine.

If foods such as turkey are so high in tyrosine, why use a supplement? There are a few reasons. One, will your child eat the exact same amount of turkey every day, at the same time of day? Do you want to prepare it daily? Does it deliver enough tyrosine to work for your child? Are you certain your child digests these foods adequately to deliver the right dose of tyrosine into the brain? It's not likely that you can answer yes to all these questions. When using an amino acid or any supplement for a therapeutic effect, consistent dosing is essential to success, just as is true for medications. A supplement permits you to easily administer and control the right dose. (In fact, when my nutrition care plans have unraveled for kids, it is often because a parent simply didn't follow instructions for consistent dosing, forgot to "refill" a supplement and continue it, bought a cheap and ineffective substitute product, or thought that because it's a nutrient, it's okay to use it inconsistently.) Another reason: Amino acids compete for absorption into the brain, where they feed neurotransmitter pathways. Protein foods have a number of amino acids in them, awaiting liberty via digestion. If you want to favor a particular amino acid for a specific purpose in brain chemistry, give it a leg up with a single larger dose, with no or few competing amino acids. Better yet, give it with a carbohydrate food such as toast and jam; a favorite fruit or fruit smoothie *without* protein powder, soy milk, or milk; or something like pumpkin bread, so that energy requirements are sure to be covered at the same time. This protects the amino acid from being cannibalized for energy, and preserves it for its duty in neurotransmitter pathways.

When a therapeutically relevant dose of tyrosine is given, within an hour children will usually experience a shift in their countenance, with more relaxed or pleasantly bouncy alertness and readiness for tasks. Watch for news from school about better performance and focus, or papers coming home that look like they were done by someone else's child because they are complete! If no change or only a small benefit is noted, then your child may need a higher dose, and may also have skipped the necessary cofactor vitamins and minerals that run neurotransmitter chemistry. Children who plainly don't need tyrosine will become agitated or too active on it; if this is the case, simply stop—it will leave your child's system in a few hours or less. Children or teens weighing over 100 pounds may need as much as 1000 milligrams of tyrosine in the morning to notice an effect (but don't start there; begin with 250 milligrams and increase as needed). You can boost the effect at lunchtime by packing high-tyrosine foods such as tofu, edamame, soy milk, hard-boiled egg or egg salad sandwich, salmon or turkey salad, avocado or guacamole dip, bananas, or almonds (if plain almonds are too boring, try seasoned ones that add a kick of spice, salt, or natural sweetener such as honey, stevia, or agave). You can also add a second smaller dose of tyrosine in your child's sack lunch by stirring it into applesauce or soft food, or mixing it into a sandwich spread.

Too Much Tyrosine?

Signs that your child has too much tyrosine are feeling agitated, anxious, restless, or jittery, rapid heartbeat or palpitations, feeling too wakeful or unable to fall asleep, or headaches. For children with autism, "stim" behaviors may worsen, along with hyperactivity and irritability. This could be helpful information for your provider team, so don't regard it as a total failure: It signals that your child's brain chemistry is possibly excessive for dopamine, which could help a prescriber choose a drug more correctly, if you've tried nutrition tools but didn't get the results you'd like. Don't use tyrosine in the evening or near bedtime, as it may make your child too wakeful. It should not be combined with psychotropic or stimulant medication, or any medications for that matter, without professional guidance. Don't add tyrosine to SSRIs, seizure medications, MAO inhibitors, or any medication without checking with your doctor first. Your child may not need tyrosine indefinitely. If its benefits seem to wane, trial a few days with no tyrosine and see how your child's mood, energy level, and work habits shift. If worse, then reintroduce it and titrate up to a slightly higher dose. Increase the dose incrementally, and use the lowest effective dose. If better, continue on the new dose for a few more weeks, but stop or lower the dose if there is new trouble sleeping or agitation. Take another break from tyrosine every few weeks to see if your child still needs it. Since tyrosine levels have been found to be elevated in melanoma, long-term use is discouraged, especially in persons with fair skin or many moles. No guidelines are officially set on this for adults or children, another reason to use tools like this with professional monitoring. Supplements that decrease tyrosine level are N-acetyl cysteine (NAC), vitamin C, vitamin E, and pyridoxal-5-phosphate (the active form of vitamin B6).

As with any supplement, quality matters. I like NOW brand tyrosine powder because it is easy to dose, reasonably priced, widely available, and effective. Whenever you buy supplements, it pays to choose a reputable supplement company's product. Choose a company that can show it uses strict and independent quality controls. It may cost more but it frequently makes the difference between an effective versus ineffective product. A helpful explanation of supplement quality standards, regulations, and seals can be found at SupplementQuality.com.

Homework: The witching hour. How many of us have struggled with our kids through tears, tantrums, or oppositional behavior when it's time for homework? How do you get a child to martial new focus in the evening, when a stimulant medication given in the morning has long since worn off? Has your child stared blankly at the papers before him, locked in confusion over what the assignment was that day? If evenings are like this in your home, try a small second dose of tyrosine after school—half of the morning dose or less. If this is too agitating and keeping your child from falling asleep, then another amino acid to consider is theanine.

Theanine is a nonessential amino acid used to increase alertness, improve memory and focus, and lessen ADHD. It is sometimes used for improving sleep as well. It does not appear to induce drowsiness. One trial showed that it improved the quality of sleep in test subjects, though they did not fall asleep faster. Theanine increases alpha brain wave activity, which is the type of activity our brains have when we are relaxed but alert at the same time, as in meditation. It may lower blood pressure, increase dopamine in the brain, and increase GABA (gamma-aminobutyric acid), all of which promote a relaxed sense of well-being. It has even been reviewed as hopeful for Alzheimer's disease, for its ability to reduce impairments in memory.

No reports of toxicity for theanine have been reported as of this writing. Both the FDA and the government in Japan, where it has been available for several more years, deem it safe. However, as with other amino acids, I rarely suggest it for children under four or five years old, simply because little is known about its use in this age group. If you want to try theanine, your child should weigh 60 pounds or more. Start with a dose of 25–50 milligrams, and stop at 100 milligrams. Children weighing 80 pounds or more should not take more than 200 milligrams of theanine without the supervision of a heath professional, such as a licensed naturopath. Purchase the "L" form (L-theanine), not the "D" form, which is a mirror image isomer molecule. Children can use a sublingual theanine spray that delivers 50 milligrams per pump, such as EndoTrex oral spray by NeuroScience. Capsules are available for older children, typically in 100-milligram doses. Try giving theanine about an hour before dinner, on an empty stomach or with a small carb snack. It is best not taken with a full meal or protein foods especially at first, to see its effect more clearly. It may help your child get his evening homework done. Experiment with dosing after dinner, too, if you like, to find the best fit.

Theanine will go to work more quickly when given with a small amount of carbohydrate food as described above, such as applesauce, fruit, a smoothie, or even an after-dinner treat. Too much may make it hard for children to fall asleep. Theanine may also be a helpful choice over tyrosine in kids who have considerable hyperactivity with inattention and lack of focus. Tyrosine may be too stimulating for these kids, while theanine may nudge them toward better focus with less mobility and energy. For these kids, a good combo may be to give at least 400 milligrams of high-quality DHA daily, with minerals as described earlier (magnesium, calcium, iron, chromium, and selenium), and theanine in the morning and after school.

More Mellowing Tools

If your child is outright anxious and stressed, emphasis on calming neurotransmitters will be important, whether you are medicating or using nutrition supports. It's important to know that chronically low total calorie intakes can worsen mood swings and anxiety in children. This can be a problem with using methylphenidate stimulant prescription medications such as Ritalin or Concerta, which may diminish appetite. Simply ensuring that your child is actually getting the calories and nutrients she needs every day can even out mood and lessen anxiety and irritability. If it's time for more targeted nutrition tools, shoring up GABA may be fruitful. Normally, GABA is the most plentiful neurotransmitter in the brain. Our understanding of its role in conditions such as autism, seizure disorders, and mood disorders is far from complete, but in each of these, too little GABA is functioning in the brain. It has an inhibitory effect on nerve cells rather than excitatory, meaning that it will generally have relaxing, antianxiety, or anticonvulsive effects. It is a relaxation chemical for the brain; when GABA is chronically depleted, we feel anxious, panicky, depressed, and stressed. Other signs are having sweaty palms and feeling clammy, feeling overwhelmed, being unable to loosen up or literally having a stiffness throughout the body; even heart palpitations and anxiety attacks can come with insufficient GABA. Drugs that treat low GABA include Valium, Xanax, or Ativan, GABA uptake inhibitors such as gabapentin or tiagabine (typically for seizure control), or benzodiazepines. Nutrients that are needed to make GABA include the right amount of B vitamins, certain amino acids (especially glutamine, and possibly theanine), zinc, and iron; herbs that are GABA inducing are valerian, bacopa, and scullcap. Mercury interferes with GABA production.

GABA has been available as an oral supplement for a long time in the United States, and it is also quite safe, but usually is used by adults and older children—again, simply because the idea of using these tools instead of prescription medications for younger children is relatively new here. In Japan, it is added to candy, soft drinks, and other foods as an antistress tool (though its efficacy in those forms is unclear). New products are emerging in the U.S. market for this same purpose. Some debate exists about which forms are most effective, and whether GABA can effectively cross the blood-brain barrier from an oral dose. GABA is often used in larger doses, even up to 3–4 grams (that's 3000–

4000 milligrams) for adults, presumably to overcome its poor up-take into the brain. GABA is mostly made *in* the brain, from raw materials present there, in neurons specifically purposed for this job—so just *eating* GABA may not be effective. Some GABA is made in the pancreas (most diabetics have antibodies to enzymes needed to make GABA, interestingly), and our adrenal glands have receptors for GABA (our adrenals sit atop our kidneys, and make stress response hormones). Whether GABA supplementation helps by trickling a bit into the brain, or through its effects on other GABA receptors elsewhere in the body, is unclear. At least one topical version (GabaMag) is available, which may be ideal for children who won't swallow a supplement in any form. Try it at bedtime to see if it assists with anxiety and sleep.

It's true that you will want to use only the lowest effective dose with any supplement, but it's especially important to do so with amino acids. These have distinct dose-specific neurotransmitter effects, unlike most vitamins, minerals, or functional nutrients such as coenzyme Q10—which may be tolerable in a wide dosage range. Small children can take a quarter or half a 100-milligram sublingual tablet (25 milligrams or 50 milligrams), depending on their weight and age, as a starting point. Several products are available that blend GABA with other calming agents such as valerian, chamomile, magnesium, or other aminos such as 5-hdyroxytrpytophan and taurine. Whatever you choose, it should show results quickly, within the first few days or sooner.

Anecdotally, oral GABA supplements seem to help some children. Data on this is scant. It is safe to use and worth a try. If your child has been taking a GABA supplement and you have not noted improvement in her anxiety, stress, or sleeplessness, stop and ask for guidance from a knowledgeable provider. You may need a different dose altogether, a different product, or a different form. Some GABA is synthetic; some is naturally produced by gut-friendly microbes such as *Lactobacillus hilgardii* (which is used to make a traditional fermented Korean dish called kimchi), and harvested for commercial use. If your child takes it in the daytime for anxiety or stress, but is becoming too sleepy then, switch to using it in the afternoon or at bedtime.

If GABA isn't easy to absorb into the brain from an oral dose, what about using glutamine, its amino acid precursor, as a supplement? Glutamine is a nonessential amino acid that occurs in many foods. It is what the brain converts to GABA, with just one biochemical jump: Glutamine becomes glutamate, which is converted to GABA. Glutamine is popular in the functional medicine and naturopathic medicine communities for gut tissue health and repair, and is often added for that purpose. But for children with autism spectrum issues, ADHD, or anxiety disorders, there is the possibility that using glutamine will backfire. Glutamate and GABA are like the yin and yang of neurotransmitters—glutamate being excitatory, and GABA calming. But in autism, emerging evidence suggests impairment in the "GABA shunt" may exist, which prevents normal balancing between these two chemicals. Too much glutamate piles up, too little GABA is created; seizures, agitation, or extreme anxiety can ensue when the balance is skewed for glutamate. This is why I generally do not use glutamine supplements for children in my caseload, even for gut tissue repair, in the context of anxiety, history of seizures, or difficulty with modulating reactivity to stress.

Instead of glutamine, there are herbal GABA uptake inhibitors that may work without ill effects. These have shown an ability to prevent too-rapid destruction of GABA between nerve cells.

Ask an experienced licensed naturopathic doctor about valerian, scullcap, or bacopa. Using these as herb tinctures or capsules may be helpful for your child. Other notable calming herbs for children are passion flower, milky oat seed, or chamomile. Very young children and toddlers can use glycerite (not alcohol) tinctures such as Sleepy Nights for Kids or Quiet Time (by WishGarden Herbs) for calming and improved sleep. Prescription GABA uptake inhibitors such as gabapentin or tiagabine are used in children for seizure control, but typically not for anxiety or stress. In kids with ADHD, abnormal glutamate function in neurons that are supposed to make dopamine is suspected. Reducing glutamine toxicity may be helpful in kids with ADHD, too.

More Tools for Calming or Anxiety

Taurine is another amino acid known for a calming effect. Anywhere from 200 to 1000 milligrams have been used in children; in fact, it is often added to infant formula, since babies may not be able to make enough of their own taurine from dietary proteins. Taurine exerts a protective effect on visual nerves in newborn rats who have seizures, and can help repair those nerves; if taurine is deficient in infancy, a long-term effect may be impaired vision. Children with autism and ADHD have been shown to lack taurine in some research. Taurine can counteract the overstimulating toxicity caused by excess glutamate at certain receptors in the brain—which means it may literally quell a too-fast electrical potentiation between nerve cells. This has long made taurine of interest to persons with epilepsy and seizure disorders. Taurine does not usually trigger sleepiness. In higher doses, it may lower blood pressure and cholesterol. Since it is needed to form bile, and bile is needed to help digest fat, there is some research showing that taurine supplements help children with cystic fibrosis absorb fat better. You can start your child with a 200-milligram dose of taurine and work up slowly. It may work best given twice daily. Don't exceed 600 milligrams per day for a toddler or 1000 milligrams per day for an older child, without expert guidance.

For a child who is easily agitated, who escalates suddenly and unpredictably into tantrums, whose parents have been told he should be on Risperdal or Abilify, or who has trouble modulating his emotional responses, consider carnosine. This is a dipeptide (two amino acids stuck together) that is plentiful in beef, chicken, and pork—another ordinary and safe compound that has neurotransmitter effects. Emerging research shows that it can oppose glutamate toxicity, just like taurine or GABA, and is thus also of growing interest to those in the epilepsy community. This "neuroprotective" effect is key to stemming a toxic surge of calcium ions through receptors in the brain, because unabated calcium flow will keep electrical potential open, resulting in seizure activity or hyperstimulation. Research shows carnosine may do this rather handily, along with controlling the flow of zinc and copper ions through nerve synapses. In practice, I have observed carnosine to improve cognition, help expressive language effort, and modulate outbursts, rage reactions, and emotional lability. Like the other calming neurotransmitters, it seems to help engage the "off" switch for children, so they may become more able to stop themselves from a roiling rage cascade. Carnosine is available as a liquid or as capsules. Start with a 250-milligram dose and work up slowly. One clinical trial used 800 milligrams per day in children with autism and saw myriad benefits in behavior, socialization, and language. Some children may need 1000 milligrams per day or higher. If given to excess, or if it is the wrong tool for a child, it may trigger hyperactivity. If you suspect this, withdraw carnosine and start over at a lower dose, or move on to other tools if even small amounts are problematic.

IS IT ANXIETY OR DEPRESSION?

It's important to get an accurate professional assessment of whether your child is managing anxiety or depression or both, before trying a nutritional or pharmaceutical intervention. For low affect with anxiety, many children are prescribed selective serotonin reuptake inhibitors (SSRIs). If you'd like to try an alternative first, 5-hydroxytryptophan (5-HTP) is a reasonable option. As with any mood disorder for a child, the basic nutrition needs should be addressed first—total calories, normal bowel function without bowel infections, and key vitamins and minerals for neurotransmitter chemistry should be on board. The next easy add-on for depression is omega-3 oils, discussed earlier; it's the omega-3 EPA (eicosapentanoic acid) that you need to add in that case, 1–3 grams per day at least. If you've been there and done all that, and your child still needs help, then you can move to the aminos for depression.

5-HTP is a widely available supplement. Not to be confused with tryptophan, it is one step away from conversion to serotonin in the brain, which is the neurotransmitter we all know and love as a modulator for mood, sleep, and appetite. SSRIs treat depression by leaving more serotonin in synapses between nerves, and preventing its destruction. Nutrition tools come at it the other way, that is, by helping you make more serotonin. 5-HTP is easily absorbed into the brain and gut, where most of our serotonin is made. Start with a 25-milligram dose and work up to 50, 100, or

150 milligrams in small increments. Do not mix 5-HTP with any medications without asking your prescriber first, or with Saint John's wort, which also impacts serotonin chemistry. You should notice a change in your child's affect within a day or two (or even within the hour), if you are using the correct dose of 5-HTP. Do not exceed 200 milligrams per day; if you are using this much, split the dose into two servings, after school and at bedtime. As with all amino acids, the effect will be clearer if given without other protein foods, so that you favor quick uptake of the dose into target tissues. In some research, 5-HTP has been shown to raise serotonin levels more than some SSRIs.

How much is too much? Whether you are using natural tools like supplements or herbs, or a prescription SSRI, you need to know that too much serotonin can be dangerous. "Serotonin syndrome" can be induced by the wrong dose of an SSRI medication or by a supplement. Its symptoms occur quickly—within a few hours or even less—when too much of a serotonin-boosting agent is given. Serotonin syndrome symptoms include chills, feeling cold, or having uncontrollable shivers; restlessness or agitation, dilated pupils, sweating, muscle twitches, rapid heart rate, goose bumps, or confusion. A severe case can be life-threatening and may trigger fainting, fever, or seizures. If you note any of these signs in your child when using an SSRI medication or a supplement, alert your doctor right away. If symptoms are worsening rapidly, go to the emergency room. Ask your doctor about giving your child activated charcoal, which may safely absorb some of the serotonin-boosting substance so your child can excrete it.

Note that children who struggle with anxiety may benefit more from serotonin boosting if it is pushed at the end of the day or bedtime, when cortisol levels are naturally dropping, rather than first thing in the morning. Cortisol is a hormone we produce in response to stress, and it is at its peak in the morning. Lots of kids with autism, ADHD, or any special need are stressed-out and chronically overproducing cortisol as a result, especially in the morning, when they may feel anticipatory anxiety about school. Mixing this with a boost to serotonin levels may worsen, not improve, anxiety. If your child tried an SSRI and became more agitated and anxious rather than less, cortisol chemistry may have been part of the puzzle. Nourishing normal cortisol levels can help children cope with stress. Gentle herbs that do this are ashwaganda, rhodiola, Holy Basil, and licorice root. These are available as capsules or tinctures. Look for reputable suppliers such as Gaia Herbs, who use careful timing when harvesting their herbs, grow them organically, and guarantee potency. One convenient product in their line is called Adrenal Health, which combines several herbs that nourish adrenal glands and mitigate stress response chemistry in the body. Rhodiola, present in this product, may also enhance dopamine, which is a plus for children needing some support for attention. Rhodiola has been extensively studied as an adaptogen, that is, as a chemical that improves the body's stress response, in part by improving our efficiency for oxygenating muscle and brain. As always, it's advisable to consult a licensed naturopath or experienced MD provider when considering these tools.

Two hundred milligrams of 5-HTP are plenty for a teenager; 100 milligrams are plenty for a school-age child. If this has no effect, consider a trial of tryptophan itself, which is one step farther removed from serotonin than 5-HTP in our biochemical machinery, or consider Saint John's wort. Don't mix serotonin boosters; use them methodically, separately, at the lowest effective dose as guided by your provider. I have not used tryptophan or Saint John's wort in practice with children, only because I have not needed to so far. The nutrition corrections described here, plus 5-HTP, have been successful for children I have worked with whose parents were looking for an alternative to SSRIs. If you would like to try tryptophan or Saint John's wort, work with a reputable supplement supplier, and a knowledgeable provider who has used these tools before in children. Tryptophan, 5-HTP, and Saint John's wort all elevate serotonin. Don't mix them, or mix them with SSRIs or other medications. Serotonin syndrome can occur when serotonin is elevated too much, causing heart palpitations, changes in blood pressure, nausea, fever, agitation, or even death. SSRIs can trigger serotonin syndrome also, which is why it is necessary to follow your prescriber's instructions when using any tool that impacts serotonin level. If your child has supplemented serotonin-boosting nutrition tools for a long stretch (six to twelve months or more) and you are not sure if they are still needed, it's easy to find out: With your provider's guidance, withdraw them at regular intervals. Amino acids are easier to discontinue than pharmaceuticals because they do not build up in your child's body as medications do. They are in and out of the metabolism much more quickly. It is not necessary to gradually reduce an amino acid dose, unless your provider directs you to do so.

If none of these tools—pharmaceutical or nutritional—seem to help your child's depression and anxiety even when it seems they should based on history, signs, and symptoms, ask your doctor to check thyroid function for your child. Your doctor may have ruled this out ahead of prescribing psychotropic medication anyway—but bear in mind that nutrition deficits can impair thyroid function in children, too. Low total calories, low total protein, and mineral deficits can especially confound thyroid function in children. Tell your doctor if you give your child ground flaxseed meal. It's a great source of fiber and healthy omega-3 fatty acids, but it may diminish the thyroid gland's ability to trap iodine if used long term at doses like 2 tablespoons or more per day. Other aids for mood and anxiety include exposure to bright light, vitamin D at 1000–5000 international units per day depending on your child's age, physical activity (which also pushes serotonin), and adequate vitamins (especially B-group) and minerals (magnesium, iron, zinc, chromium, and selenium).

Anxiety and obsessive-compulsive features (OCD). Many of the tools described here may lower anxiety or OCD features in children. Another that deserves mention is inositol, a sugar-alcohol found in many foods, and made from glucose in our own cells. When we have healthy bowel bacteria, one of their jobs is to produce inositol as a by-product of digesting the foods we eat—and this is perhaps yet another reason why correcting bowel flora in children with conditions like autism or ADHD improves behavior and mood. Inositol has myriad functions in the body. Lower than normal levels have been noted in the cerebrospinal fluid of those with depression. It has shown effectiveness in a number of trials for improving depression, treating OCD, and reducing panic attacks; this may be because it appears to act a bit like a serotonin reuptake inhibitor. It has very low toxicity, is safe to try even in younger children, and can be combined with other supplements or even medications (but as always, tell your health care provider before introducing it).

Inositol is used in much larger amounts than the aminos, or

than vitamins and minerals. Clinical trials review dosages of up to 18 *grams* (not milligrams) per day in adults—this may be more than a tablespoon of powder per day, depending on the product formulation. Luckily, inositol is a plain white powder with little taste—if anything, it tastes slightly sweet. It is easy to mix in soft foods or drinks. Children can start with a 1-gram (1000-milligram) dose and increase only to the smallest amount needed for effectiveness; children with OCD may need a higher dose for a good result than kids with depression or anxiety. One trial testing inositol in children with autism used a dose of 200 milligrams per kilogram per day (about 5 grams for a child who weighs 50–60 pounds), and reported no benefit; this study had only nine test subjects. Another tested myoinositol on seizure activity in rats, and found it significantly reduced seizures. The therapeutic range for adults is 12–18 grams per day; I once used 4 grams with beneficial results in a three-year-old who was advised to use medication for anxiety by a top neurologist. Products like True Hope Inositol give 1000 milligrams per quarter teaspoon. Young teens may need an adult dose for efficacy, which can be spaced out in two or three doses after lunchtime. Inositol can make you sleepy, or trigger nausea or gas in larger doses. It may be best used near bedtime for this reason. For kids who are especially anxious about going to school, it can work well to give it in the morning. See the resources section for a favorite morning smoothie for many kids in my practice, who have food allergies, need a calorie boost, and need calming before school.

Inositol will typically work quickly if benefits are to be had. William Walsh, PhD, of the Pfeiffer Treatment Center in Illinois finds that inositol works well in kids and adults who have OCD, high histamine levels, and depleted methylation chemistry, but poorly in those with overmethylated brain pathways. These are specific nutritional biochemistries that providers in integrative psychiatry can assess. His clinic and others that follow alternative treatments in psychiatry claim success in running lab tests on clients first to determine these factors before prescribing any nutrients or medications. Visit the website of the American Psychiatric Association Caucus on Complementary, Alternative, and Integrative Care (APACAM.org) or the Pfeiffer Treatment Center's site (HRIPTC.org) for more information on assessing and treating psychiatric disorders with complementary medicine tools.

Neurotransmitter Cofactors

Amino acids are needed by the brain to build neurotransmitters, while certain vitamins and minerals are needed to put those amino acids together in the right sequences. This is why it's so important to thoughtfully supplement children trying amino acids with the right doses of vitamins and minerals if they aren't eating a varied enough diet to get these daily, and/or can't absorb them very well. Most children in my practice do not! Vitamin and mineral cofactors engage at the right moment in cell chemistry—almost as the moving parts of a kinetic sculpture will do, to move balls along or ring chimes—so that the process to make neurotransmitters can run smoothly. For neurotransmitter chemistry, B vitamins and certain minerals (copper, iron, manganese, molybdenum, and magnesium) are especially important. It's no coincidence that high doses of B-group vitamins have long been favored to intervene for stress—but this will mean little for a child who can't effectively extract amino acids from food proteins to begin with, who eats a diet with a low total protein intake, or who has weak mineral status.

Pyridoxine (vitamin B6) and its active form (pyridoxal-5-phosphate, or P5P) are especially pertinent to producing serotonin, dopamine, epinephrine, and norepinephrine. Pyridoxine was one of the first nutrients considered for conditions such as autism and schizophrenia, back in the 1960s. Is it effective to add only B vitamins, or other vitamins and minerals, while changing nothing else in your child's food intake or nutrition plan? I do meet parents who are so averse to dietary or other total nutrition measures that they simply add supplements for their children in hopes of seeing big shifts. Others will begin with a high dose of B6 to see if anything will change, since this is easy to add and has very low toxicity. Unless a child has mild or nearly typical needs, I do not usually witness a dramatic or sustainable improvement with this approach. As always, exactly how supplements should be added depends on the child's needs, which are best assessed professionally. For children, this means reviewing growth data, food intake data, medical history, signs and symptoms that are notoriously peculiar to B vitamin deficits, and lab data. Lab data alone isn't the whole story when assessing B vitamin status in kids. If your provider has run a battery of tests only to declare that you need to buy a bunch of supplements, don't be surprised if this doesn't solve all your child's problems—levels of certain B vitamins in blood don't necessarily reflect the functional status of this nutrient, and no blood test can assess total food intakes in kids, a key piece in understanding child nutrition status.

Labs reviewing B vitamin status should also consider red blood cell status, since B vitamins are needed for normal red blood cell formation. This can be reviewed with an ordinary test any pediatrician can order called a CBC, or complete blood count. A CBC counts and differentiates red and white blood cells; when certain nutrients are lacking (from poor intake, malabsorption, or both), blood cells yield telltale signs on this test. Urine organic acid testing that reflects uptake of B vitamins into cells may be helpful, too—in particular, a parameter called methylmalonic acid (MMA), which is measurable in blood or urine, can infer whether or not your child might be a responder to methylcobalamin therapy. Methylcobalamin is the methylated form of vitamin B12 that has triggered dramatic improvements for some children with autism, ADD, or ADHD. Therapeutic protocols use injected or inhaled forms of this vitamin, prescribed by a knowledgeable physician. Finally, good clinicians will know about classic signs and symptoms in children that suggest poor status for certain B vitamins. Let an experienced provider support your efforts here. Meanwhile, you can supplement your child with a basic multivitamin that gives a good complement of the entire B complex (thiamine, niacin, riboflavin, cobalamin, pantothenic acid, folic acid, pyridoxine, and biotin).

Using very high doses of B vitamins and of pyridoxine in particular (vitamin B6) can be stimulating or agitating. Don't give B vitamins at bedtime; if you give your child melatonin for sleep, be sure you use a product that doesn't add B6, as some do. Some products for children with autism offer absolutely astronomical doses of B vitamins. I have not usually found these to be necessary, once bowel infections, overall nutrient status, and food intakes are improved. If you are using high-dose Bs and your child has hyperactivity or reactivity, take a supplement holiday and assess if this is the right product to use. It may work better to introduce a different product at a lower dose, or to switch to a topical B complex cream, which is great for kids with malabsorption. B vitamins are generally easy to trial, because of their low toxicity. Some very sensitive children may have spikes in agitation or hyperactivity with high-dose Bs, so start with a low dose and work up slowly to see if any benefit might be had.

There are many miles to go before we can claim to comprehend neurotransmitter chemistry in full, or say we know with certainty how to best redirect it for children suffering with anxiety, depression, bipolar disorder, OCD, autism, ADHD, and so on. What *is* clear is that drugs are not the only answer for all children. A standout example was documented by Andrew Stoll, MD, from Harvard, on using high-dose omega-3 fatty acids (9 grams per day) to treat bipolar disorder. Other compelling research exists on the success of naturopathic tools for these concerns— whether you consider them instead of, before, after, or even with pharmaceuticals for your child. Other options not mentioned here include treatment to remove heavy metal toxins such as lead and mercury, which impair cognition and derail many neurotransmitter pathways, herbs from the realms of Ayurvedic or Chinese medicine, and homeopathic remedies. In Boulder, where I live, it's easy to find practitioners with expertise in complementary disciplines, and most major metropolitan areas offer this. If you can't find the providers you need in your own community, contact national organizations representing their disciplines, and ask for referrals.

Chapter Six

Beyond the Pediatrician

GOING PHARM-FREE WITH
MORE RESOURCES AND EXPERTS

What can families do when their pediatricians have run out of answers? I meet many parents who have faced this question. What if:

- Your child's chronic condition has not improved or has improved only marginally under the guidance, care, or referrals offered by your pediatrician.

- You are interested in weaning your child off medications, but your pediatrician isn't able to guide you on alternatives to laxatives, psychotropic medications, anti-inflammatories, steroids, statins, or reflux medications (each of which may have costly nutritional impacts when used long term).

- You have concerns about the vaccination schedule your pediatrician wants you to follow.

- You have been told you will have to leave your pediatrician's practice if you don't vaccinate as directed.

- You would like a health care strategy for your child that is more holistic and integrative, and less dependent on pharmaceuticals.

Each of these scenarios has been lamented to me by distraught parents. They are valid reasons to part company with a professional you need to entrust with the well-being of your children, and find more workable options. I am often asked to suggest pediatric practices that allow flexibility on vaccination schedules. You can explore this by visiting AskDrSears.com, a site by pediatric physician specialists William, James, and Robert Sears, all MDs with stellar credentials in practice, parenting, and publishing. This site includes a page called "What is a vaccine-friendly doctor?" which answers the many questions parents have about this. The vaccination schedule has become increasingly crowded in the last twenty years with over fifty vaccines now given to U.S. children in the first years of life; this continues to coincide with increases in autism, infant mortality rates, and other chronic disabilities and diseases. A recent survey of more than 1,500 parents found that over one-fourth of them believe that vaccines can trigger autism. With virtually no pediatricians agreeing with them, it's easy to see why this family-provider relationship is crumbling. Compelling research has raised concerns about the impact of the full vaccine schedule on children, relative to developmental outcomes, asthma, allergies, seizure disorders, and even diabetes.* This is politically volatile territory. With our pediatricians and vaccine manufacturers enjoying federal protection from liability for any negative effects from vaccines, some argue that they are too removed from these impacts—and too close to the financial reward that vaccines provide—to clearly judge.

No matter what your position is on the vaccine controversy, you can still leverage pharmaceutical alternatives that have a track record for infection fighting, nutritional replenishment, and regulating mood or focus. But who is the expert in the know? Many parents wonder where to turn to augment the pediatrician's expertise. There are, in fact, many other places to turn. In my role as a registered dietitian, I review all kinds of other providers' input when doing nutrition assessments on babies and kids. I read everything from endoscopy reports to swallow studies, from NICU notes and speech and language assessments to individualized education plans (IEPs); from endocrinology consult letters between physicians to all sorts of lab data from naturopaths, when piecing together nutrition care plans. These documents come from files of children in most every U.S. state and a number of other countries. What amazes me most about this is witnessing the great lengths and expense parents go to for health care that isn't creating the progress their children need. The kids with the thickest

* For a list of lesser-known studies that have found safety concerns with vaccinations, go to FourteenStudies.org. Visit SafeMinds.org for analysis of conflicts of interest and methodology deficits in research currently used to exonerate vaccines. Some studies showing vaccine safety concerns are also available at my site, NutritionCare.net.

files are usually the ones making the least progress—not because of any neglect on their parents' part, but because of ineffective or poorly coordinated care tools from the medical profession.

Typically, by the time parents come into my office, they have already searched beyond the pediatrician. They've seen various pediatric medical specialists, which in many cases involved getting in an airplane to travel to an appointment. They are weary. They have had to give the speech they are about to give me on their children's history a lot, perhaps dozens of times. They have become efficient in this dreary task, toting organized notebooks full of lab data, growth charts, and progress notes. It's not unusual for parents to hand me tabulated binders with sections organized for allergy, neurology, occupational therapy, endocrinology, general pediatric visits, and so on. They've run the gamut of conventional pediatrics and pushed the limits of what's allowable in their insurance networks for specialists. But their kids are still not growing, not developing typically, not eating more than three foods, not able to function in a classroom. Their kids' needs simply weren't met by conventional pediatric medicine. They are at their wit's end by the time they enter my office.

As you might have guessed by now, usually no one has looked too closely at the nutrition piece of the puzzle for these kids. If it *has* been looked at, it was often with a glancing nod by a hospital dietitian who couldn't help much, or by a provider in another discipline who respects nutrition but has no particular training in it relative to infants and children. Oftentimes, the parent has decided to tackle the nutrition piece alone, and has placed the child on an inadequate, ineffective diet with supplements that aren't helpful either. These meandering approaches to such a pivotal piece can make for lousy results, and will lead many doctors to wave nutrition off entirely as fringe (even though it *is* a science grounded in decades of evidence-based findings). Unless the dietitian you talk to works in a hospital, nutrition care isn't considered "medical" either—which is strange, because it requires the same standardized degree of training, hundreds of hours of supervised clinical rotations, a hefty exam, and professionally monitored continuing education to be a registered dietitian or licensed nutrition professional, no matter where you work. But like a lot of doctors in hospitals, dietitians there don't implement complementary and alternative approaches either, because it's not what the hospital is under contract to deliver (thank your health insurer for that).

While medical practice is frequently divided by anatomy (for example, neurology, gastroenterology, nephrology, cardiology), nutrition is more often divided into specialization by life stages, conditions, or functions: There are registered dietitians and licensed nutrition professionals who specialize in pediatrics, geriatrics, maternal health and prenatal nutrition, sports and fitness, diabetes, weight management, oncology, eating disorders, and so on. A neurologist can do a brain scan, and will consider surgeries or medications for the brain. A gastroenterologist can look at parts of the digestive system, and will apply medications or procedures to treat those parts. Allergists will focus mostly on lungs and skin with prescription medications. But nutrition goes to all cells, everywhere. Working with this requires me to be a generalist; I must consider how nutrients impact every body part, not just one organ. This approach often triggers shifts for children that weren't obtained with the parade of specialists, simply because we focus on problems that were overlooked, and we connect the body parts into one system rather than several separate systems. This is a big "we," because while I may be a guide, the parents do most of the work. Their success often triggers curiosity about other integrative modalities that do this, too: homeopathy, naturopathic care, traditional Chinese medicine, or chiropractic care—things that may make a pediatrician roll his eyes in skeptical disapproval!

This is already starting to change. Collaborative efforts between conventional medical care tools and what are now considered "alternative" are increasing. In 2002, the White House Commission on Complementary and Alternative Medicine Policy presented recommendations to the president on an appropriate blueprint for increasing access to safe and effective complementary medicine. Congress had already established the National Center for Complementary and Alternative Medicine in 1998, within the National Institutes of Health. Its mission is to fund research on alternative medicine and provide training in it as well. Alternative medicine tools are in full swing in most other industrialized countries, where parents often take it for granted that finding what works for a child's health is not an either/or proposition. It's not about whether you go to a conventional pediatrician or not, or a chiropractor or not, or a homeopath or not; in many countries, these are all part of the health care system.

Reputable providers of complementary and alternative therapies know the value of conventional medical tools, and direct patients to them accordingly. This is a "whatever works" situation, and what works is not necessarily *only* to be found in your pediatrician's or MD specialist's office. What works may be some combination of tools, modalities, and providers that you feel comfortable with; perhaps there is an array of tools that can benefit your child. You are a health consumer on your child's behalf, and can choose safe alternatives that work. If your child is not attaining the health she deserves, feel free to explore beyond what your in-network MD has offered, by seeking out other experts. Having shared case notes with physicians across the continent now for years, I have found that MDs who are confident in their science and practice are frequently open to modalities they have not been trained in. As long as a child is progressing well with no harm done, they often become supportive.

This approach to child health is big in Boulder, Colorado, where companies such as Pharmaca are thriving. Pharmaca is an "integrative" pharmacy with stores in Western states. On duty in any Pharmaca store at any time is a pharmacist to work with your physician, answer questions about medications, and fill prescriptions. You will also find a certified homeopath or licensed naturopathic doctor walking the aisles to help with purchases and answer questions, plus a broad array of medicinal herbs, supplements, and homeopathic remedies for sale right alongside the usual ibuprofen, Band-Aids, or milk of magnesia. Literally, conventional and complementary medicine tools share shelf space—they are integrated under one roof. Consumer demand for this integrative approach is spreading. Referred to as "CAM" in the medical literature (for complementary and alternative medicine), it has been found to be increasingly popular according to many surveys. Here's an introduction to four CAM modalities that more parents are exploring—and having success with—for their kids than ever before.

Homeopathy

What *is* this modality that enjoys more acceptance elsewhere in the world—especially in Germany, France, India, and the United

Kingdom—than it does in the United States? In France, homeo-pathics are dispensed in state pharmacies; taught in schools of dentistry, pharmacy, veterinary, and midwifery; and covered by state insurance. In England, the royal family has famously relied on homeopathy for decades. It is a covered national health option, and nearly half of all British physicians refer patients for this type of care, despite regular and organized opposition from pharma-ceutical interest groups. A number of British hospitals practice homeopathy and have waiting lists for homeopathic treatment appointments. In India, even Gandhi endorsed its use despite his own country's well-respected 5,000-year-old tradition of Ay-urvedic medicine. In Germany, surveys indicate that over a third of their physicians prescribe homeopathy. CAM is so popular there that training to practice it is mandated for all physicians. More endorsements for homeopathy are found around the world, from Switzerland to Asia.

For all its supporters, homeopathy has no shortage of un-abashed detractors, who insist that it is a sham modality that elic-its only placebo effects. This argument is based on the fact that homeopathic medicines have no detectable therapeutic sub-stance in them. Made from all manner of materials—from miner-als to plants and animals to diseased human tissue—homeopathic remedies are prepared through a series of dilutions of these ma-terials that are agitated, shaken, or stirred at each dilution. Once the desired potency is reached, the dilution is then made into tiny sugar pellets that melt on the tongue, or as drops in purified water. The more dilute the remedy, the more potent its effect—a paradox that defies the very essence of conventional medical thought. Be-cause of that inexplicable paradox, many medical scientists refuse to consider research on homeopathy at all, even when methods follow Western medicine's scientific process and when the findings are statistically significant.

In curiously dissonant thinking, these are scientists who would likely applaud the same research if it showed homeopathy to be an outright hoax. That hasn't quite occurred. Some studies *have* illustrated significant benefits from homeopathy in conditions such as the flu, infections, childhood illnesses, depression and anxiety disorders, traumatic injuries, and more. Impressive case examples also abound worldwide. What really throws the conventional medical crowd is that, if it does work, nobody can really explain how or why. Some authors have attempted this. They invoke quantum theory, and proffer that the molecular signature of a substance is amplified when prepared in a series of dilutions and "succussions," as all the shaking and banging is called. Perhaps quantum physics *is* the only way to explain, in a physical sense, why homeopathy may work. In any case, if homeopathy is quantum physics in action as a healing tool, that sheds some light on why medicine—as it's taught at places like Harvard or Columbia University—can't describe what it does in the body. We have no way to measure that—not yet anyway. But we can measure before and after effects, and this is what looks favorable in some stringent trials with homeopathy.

It's a striking irony that homeopathy is based on essentially the same premise that Western medicine uses in vaccination. Its premise is "like cures like." For example, if you want to avoid the flu, your doctor offers you a flu vaccine. The vaccine contains partial information about the flu virus, just enough to make your immune system "think" you've been exposed—but you don't get sick (not usually anyway, though reports of full-blown flu after vaccination exist). A fraction of the triggering substance—the virus itself—is used to prevent the infection. Homeopathy works in a similar fashion, albeit at levels we don't know how to observe or detect. An infinitesimal amount of triggering substance is given to elicit a healing response from the body, under the same "like cures like" premise. If you are in the early stages of coming down with the flu, a homeopathic prescriber might give you a remedy made from flu virus called Oscillococcinum. A double-blind, placebo-controlled trial with this remedy showed that it triggered a statistically significant reduction in severity and duration of flu symptoms, compared to placebo. That is, users in the early stages of the flu had a shorter, milder course of infection when given this homeopathic remedy, compared to placebo.

In homeopathy, the "like cures like" premise is always applied. Homeopaths working with children are often interested in side effects or injuries from vaccines, so they may use remedies based on vaccine ingredients. For example, symptoms of mercury poisoning may be treated by a remedy made from mercury (which contains no detectable mercury). Cold symptoms such as stinging, watery eyes with clear, burning nasal mucus might be treated with a remedy made from onion, which will trigger those symptoms in a healthy person exposed to raw onion. The same cold in another child may call for a remedy made from a different substance, if the symptoms are different: A cold presenting with a teary, clingy disposition in the child, thick green nasal mucus, stinging throat, and unproductive cough might call for Pulsatilla, a remedy made from a traditional European medicinal plant called pasqueflower. Given to an infection-free person, Pulsatilla might trigger some of these symptoms.

There are hundreds of homeopathic remedies, and while it's

safe and easy to learn about a few of them to have on hand in a home first aid kit, it's best to work with trained professionals to treat illnesses in children. Certified classical homeopaths (CCHs) are trained to prescribe remedies acutely (for transient concerns, injuries, or illnesses) and constitutionally. Constitutional prescribing is for entrenched chronic conditions—such as allergies, autism, sleep problems, cancer, developmental concerns, mood disorders, emotional issues, and so on. This should definitely be left to a professional homeopath. Prescribing homeopathic remedies correctly is arguably more an esoteric art than a science. Getting it right can be dramatically successful. Getting it wrong will usually mean it doesn't help you much. In some cases, a prescription misfire can trigger unwanted side effects, just as can happen in Western medicine. Here are two examples of constitutional treatments in children—unsuccessful and successful—I've encountered:

- A potty-trained and well child age five years was given a remedy called Belladonna for anxiety and fear. This child had never wet the bed; it had never been a concern for the family, had never been discussed in front of the child, or mentioned in the child's history for the homeopath. One of Belladonna's symptoms in young children is bed-wetting. With this dose, the child began wetting the bed nightly and didn't stop for four months. The child's anxiety did not improve. This is an example of how homeopathic remedies, when chosen *incorrectly*, can produce symptoms of the remedy in healthy individuals. This peculiarity of homeopathy weakens the argument of a placebo effect, since unknown, unwanted side effects can occur.

- A child age three who was suspected of mercury toxicity from vaccinations was given a constitutional dose of Mercurius vivus, a remedy based on mercury. He had delayed social skills and couldn't tolerate being with peers. Within a few hours of receiving the dose, he went from being entirely well to spiking a high fever (104 degrees). A full body rash also bloomed quickly, starting at his head and moving downward. Both cleared in less than eighteen hours, before he got to see his pediatrician, who was contacted immediately to see the situation. By the time the boy got to the pediatric visit, the fever was resolved, the rash was nearly gone, and he was already too well for any diagnosis to be made. After fully recovering twenty-four hours later, the boy began playing and socializing normally with peers for the first time.

The example of the three-year-old above illustrates what homeopaths recognize as a "healing crisis"—that is, the body's forceful reaction to a correctly dosed remedy. When parents are accustomed to medications that mask and suppress symptoms, it can be alarming to see a child suddenly shift into what indeed looks like a crisis or worsening symptom picture. A trained homeopath will be pleased with a response like this in many cases. It signals an initiation of a healing mechanism and usually precedes strong, positive shifts. Let a certified classical homeopath guide you with dosing instructions through it, along with advice on including your pediatrician in the process.

For straightforward minor or acute conditions such as fevers, scrapes, bangs and bruises, routine illnesses, ear infections, frights, colic, or any of the usual lumps and bumps of childhood, there are several famously effective remedies. Health food stores and pharmacies alike will usually stock Arnica for injuries (as ointment or sublingual pellets) or Oscillococcinum for flu. If you're not sure whether these are right for you, talk to the pharmacist or staff at retailer locations, or consult a homeopath. Remedies for chronic issues—say, digestive problems such as diarrhea, constipation, food allergies, reflux, bloating, gas, or colic—are many. Have a homeopath review your child's case and choose a remedy for her. If your child is quickly losing fluids from vomiting and diarrhea, call your doctor or go to the emergency room. Your child may need intravenous fluids. Signs that these are needed are skin that dents and doesn't bounce back when touched, cool and pale peripheries, dizziness and lethargy, reduced urine output, and a sunken appearance to eyes. If you note these in your child, get medical attention immediately.

From teething, colic, and ear infections, to acne and distractibility in puberty, homeopathy claims victories of all sorts for children. A useful home care book is *Everybody's Guide to Homeopathic Medicines* by Stephen Cummings, MD, and Dana Ullman, MPH. This book tells you which remedies treat transient, minor, and acute conditions, so you can have these remedies on hand just as you keep cotton balls, Band-Aids, and Vaseline in the medicine cabinet. It also gives a clear delineation between when it's appropriate to use a homeopathic remedy and when it's necessary to call your doctor. This book has saved my own family many trips to the doctor's office, and afforded us many swift recoveries from minor afflictions as well as some more serious ones.

Homeopathy has become more popular for children with special needs, especially as an alternative to psychotropic medications. Homeopathic alternatives to drug treatments for Asperger's syndrome, ADHD, autism, anxiety and mood disorders, and other constitutional problems are detailed in books listed in the resources section. Don't tinker with constitutional homeopathic treatments for these conditions; consult a homeopath experienced in working with children. Research on them is scant for now, but likely to grow.

What type of training do homeopaths get? This is not a regulated field, so it is important to know what to look for. I asked Barbara Seideneck, founder and director of Homeopathy School International. Five hundred hours of training are a minimum requirement to obtain a certificate of classical homeopathy. Higher levels of training and certification can be pursued beyond this. Look for a homeopath who is either board certified or a certified classical homeopath or who is actively involved in continuing education. Board certification in homeopathy is available to MD physicians.

Chiropractic for Kids? It's "Not Just Little Spines"

Some might say that there has been a long and rather chilly relationship between medical doctors and chiropractors, and many people will be ready to share a story, true or not, of either a brilliant cure rendered by a chiropractor or a terrible injury. But when I visited with Dr. Elizabeth Decker, a chiropractor who specializes in treating women in pregnancy, infants, and children, I came away energized by the level of professionalism and passion she brings to her work. Like nutrition or any other health care modality administered to children, chiropractic care for kids differs from chiropractic care for adults. "They're not just little spines," she explained as she shared information on what this modality is. Here's what you need to know about considering chiropractic care for your special-needs infant or child:

Chiropractic care is the practice of adjusting the spine so that all nerves that travel through it (and all our nerves *do* travel through it from the brain to organs, muscles, and peripheries) can function freely, normally, and as intended. When they are injured, compressed, inflamed, or traumatized, nerves don't transmit impulses smoothly or correctly. This may manifest in children in many ways, from hyperactivity and hypersensitivities of all sorts, to low tone and floppiness, to disturbances in organ functions, or motor, cognitive, or sleep problems. The delicate structures of the spine and cranium may be susceptible to subluxations—or misalignments that alter nerve function—from physical as well as chemical traumas, or even chronic emotional stress. From carrying a heavy backpack every day to tilting one's chin into a cell phone to slouching with a laptop or computer game for hours after school, it's easy to see how mechanical issues can impede optimal alignment of vertebrae in the spine and neck. Birth traumas can contribute as well, not to mention falls, seizures, or injuries—but Dr. Decker gave some other interesting examples that particularly stand out for special-needs kids.

For example, young infants are supposed to spend a lot of time on their tummies. When they do this, they soon gain the strength to lift their heads, then push up from their palms on the floor, then curl their necks and spines as they lift their gazes to look around. Eventually, this allows a natural and necessary curvature to develop in the neck. When our necks have this curve, which is obvious on an X-ray, our necks are better shock absorbers than when these vertebrae stay straight. A "straight" neck also puts more pressure on the dura (the leather-like enclosure around the brain and spinal cord) and on the cervical vertebrae (the bones in the neck); this pressure may impede how nerves leaving the neck transmit information to the brain and body. How many parents of children with special needs watched their babies recoil from this early motor tasking, or skip it altogether? Infants who avoid tummy time are likely to experience motor delays in lifting their heads and rolling or righting themselves; if they pass over crawling, they are deleting parts of a critical sequence that let them acquire typical sensory-motor skills later on. Restoring the natural curvature of the cervical vertebrae may help children with special needs improve functional abilities on many levels, at any age. Dr. Decker also stressed how important crawling is as a developmental stage to help muscles, bones, and information processing in the brain develop typically. Chiropractors, she said, can identify where along the spine impingements may be occurring and suggest exercises children can do at home with parents and caregivers to improve nerve function, and thus the function of all the body.

A review of safety and efficacy of chiropractic care for children from 2009 found that out of more than 5,400 visits among nearly 600 children, only three "aggravations" occurred, that is, minor discomfort after the treatment. In each case, these were resolved with chiropractic care. Parents sought care for their children for muscle complaints, as well as ear, nose, throat, respiratory, and digestive conditions. They reported improved sleep patterns, immune function, behavior, and improvements in the children's presenting complaints.

What kinds of problems respond to chiropractic care in kids? Though chiropractors are treating only the spine, correcting how it is situated may improve colic, frequent ear infections, poor appetite, allergies, hyperactivity, bed-wetting, problems with focus and attention, sensory integration disorder, or other common childhood problems. When I asked Dr. Decker about seizures, she explained that she does treat some children with seizure disorders, but none who are not on medications for seizure control. Children with Down's syndrome require special techniques, owing to the hypermobility of their joints in general and in the neck in particular. Infants can be treated as well, and in her practice, she stated that spinal adjustments are so gentle, babies frequently sleep through them.

Adjustments in pediatric chiropractic are exceedingly subtle; they differ from techniques used on adults. Dr. Decker explained that there is no audible "crack" when adjusting infants and children. She may use only fingertips or just her pinkie finger with light vibration or wiggling at a point that needs adjusting, and will only treat the point that needs it. Her practice offers specialized equipment to softly cradle infants, and small adjustment tables to accommodate young children correctly. She asserted that it is important for anyone practicing chiropractic on children to be trained in that specialty. Chiropractors can be trained by certificate and diplomate programs offered by the International Chiropractic Pediatric Association; these are rigorous, requiring a minimum of 180 hours of specialized training on top of the chiropractic degree, peer-reviewed written work, and qualifying exams. Visit their website at ICPA4Kids.org for more information or to locate a qualified family practice chiropractor in your area.

Naturopathic Doctors

A naturopath is a doctor who uses only "natural" substances such as foods, supplements, or herbs to treat conditions. Some also use homeopathic remedies (though for constitutional prescribing, a certified classical homeopath is best consulted). They don't refute the efficacy of pharmaceuticals; they simply train in the use of other tools. A good naturopath has no beef with prescription medications or surgical procedures, and will refer a patient on where appropriate, while a medical doctor is not as likely to know the value of the naturopath's tools and will typically not refer a patient for an "alternative" treatment. Naturopaths must be licensed to practice in fifteen states; in all states, they must maintain proof of continuing education on an annual basis. Naturopathic doctors complete a four-year graduate course of study, a certain number of supervised clinic hours, and board exams. Residency training is not required to get an ND degree, but these are available and popular with most students working toward this degree. There are seven accredited naturopathic medical colleges in the United States.

You can obtain regular family health care with a naturopath, including routine physicals and checkups. Some naturopaths share a practice with MDs, and foster relationships with the MD community so that your family has coverage at local acute care facilities if necessary. Like family practice MDs, naturopathic doctors who work with families may be less linked up with pediatric referral specialists or Early Intervention Program services than a conventional pediatrician. If you use a naturopath as your primary pediatric provider, don't hesitate to ask about resources for occupational, speech, or behavior therapies if you need them.

Traditional Chinese Medicine

As it happens, I share office space with two practitioners of traditional Chinese medicine (TCM). One of them, Stephan, also happens to be a pediatric occupational therapist who has worked with children of all ages and presentations of special needs in a pediatric hospital. Stephan also provides acupuncture in another outpatient setting, affiliated with the same hospital network, for cancer patients. The other, Kate, works part-time as an ICU nurse. This illustrates the diverse and blended backgrounds that complementary and alternative medicine practitioners can bring to their work. Kate and Stephan exemplify health care providers who have conventional medical training as well as training and experience with an "alternative," and they still use *both*—there is no inherent conflict. They are the type of integrated practitioners that more and more families are seeking out for care.

Though I have long been an ardent fan of TCM for myself— for everything from sports injuries to insomnia—I did not know it was applied much for children here in the United States, even though (obviously) it have been used for thousands of years for children in China. Infants and children can use Chinese herbs that are formulated specifically for them in drops or tinctures. My office mates keep a pharmacy room of Chinese herbs that they prescribe, as pills, powders, or tinctures. Other TCM practitioners will use raw herbs and send patients home with instructions on how to cook them, that is, use them as "tea" (which is simply the raw herb steeped per the provider's instructions). For children, this is an improbable option (the "teas" usually taste terrible), making ready-made products preferable. Though these are often sold in stores, it is best to defer self-treatment, and consult a trained, licensed provider. Herbs can be powerful medicines and should be managed by a provider credentialed and experienced in their use, not a vitamin store clerk. TCM practitioners are monitored by state laws and professional credentialing agencies such as the National Certification Commission for Acupuncture and Oriental Medicine. Only two states, Oklahoma and Wyoming, have no laws that regulate acupuncture or TCM practice. Laws vary in other states regarding who is allowed to practice acupuncture and Oriental medicine, and how practice is monitored. In the United States, there are several accredited programs for training in Oriental medicine and acupuncture. Look for a provider who has a master's degree in acupuncture *and* Oriental medicine (not just acupuncture), as well as extensive experience and background with children in practice. Training in acupuncture and Oriental medicine assures that your provider knows how to prescribe Chinese herbs safely and effectively, while training in acupuncture only does not. In some states, medical doctors and other health care practitioners can obtain a license to practice this discipline with lesser training.

Like those who practice nutrition care, homeopathy, and chiropractic, a TCM provider will be interested in your child's physical *and* emotional complaints. Of all the modalities discussed here, TCM is probably the most different from Western medicine. Its goal is balance between what it regards as the five major organ systems, and these don't entirely correspond to our Western anatomical organ structures. In TCM, each organ system is thought to either give or drain away energy from the other four, so illnesses are considered to be an expression of weak or excessive energy patterns within those systems. This is a downright blasphemous oversimplification, but suffice it to say that herbs plus acupuncture are used to manipulate and balance these energy flows, called the meridians, on the body. Either tool given alone is usually less effective.

Families can expect to find treatments for the usual childhood problems with TCM: ear infections, colds, flu, GI concerns and colic, sprains, and pains. What about special-needs situations? It's intriguing that although TCM is one of the oldest, longest-practiced modality for medicine on earth, it has no description for autism, lending weight to the theory that this is a disease of modern toxicity overload. TCM does acknowledge developmental delays in walking, standing, hair growth, teeth eruption, and speech, and has treatment strategies for these. Other conditions, such as diabetes, are acknowledged in ancient TCM teaching (as *xiao ke*, or "wasting thirst" syndrome); a number of Chinese herbs have shown some efficacy for improving blood sugar control, with research into European blueberry, bitter melon, onion, garlic, fenugreek, ginkgo biloba, berberine, and ginseng showing some promise. That said, *if* you superimpose your child's Western diagnostic labels on Chinese medicine, you won't get very far. These don't bring much to the treatment path for a TCM practitioner, who will use traditional Chinese measures to assess the flow of life force between organ systems. While this may sound like pure "woo" to many Western medical providers, they probably don't know that training in acupuncture is currently available for physicians as a nine-month course of study at Harvard Medical School!

Homeopathy, chiropractic, naturopathics, and Oriental medicine are just four of many modalities available from the CAM landscape. More and more providers are interested in helping infants and children with these tools. It is devastating that in this era, our children are so heavily saddled with chronic disease and disability. They are expected to live shorter, less healthy lives than we are enjoying as their parents. I couldn't do my job if I couldn't find a silver lining in this, and I think it is this: Our children's urgent needs are forcing a shift in medicine. They are call-ing for an integration of old thinking with new, a blending of some tried-and-true medical skills with promising "alternative" tools that are already more widely accepted across the globe than here in the United States. See the next chapter for suggestions on working with just one sliver of this—supplements—and the resources section for more ideas on where to look for CAM supports.

Chapter Seven

Nutrition-Focused Tools 101

KNOW BEFORE YOU BUY

Using nutrition-focused tools boils down to two tasks: eating food that nurtures and promotes health, and using supplements that may benefit your children. Paying equal attention to both is necessary to really succeed, if you want to improve your children's health with these tools. Supplements won't overcome a regular diet of lousy food, and a "perfect" food intake (whatever that is) won't change the fact that your child may need anti-inflammatory supports or has dyslexia that can be lessened with targeted use of specific nutrients. Striking a balance with both is where you can get some traction to help your children feel and function better.

First, about food: Much is being discussed, blogged, and written lately about our corporate food infrastructure. Who would have thought that bestselling books could cover topics such as following the components of a meal from farm to table (*The Omnivore's Dilemma*), or how genetic modifications are spliced into the cereal or tomatoes you feed your kids (*Unhealthy Truth*)? Books such as these are popular not only because they are great reads, but because parents are reawakening to the importance of food and feeling anew the desire to shoulder the job of family wellness once and for all. We've had two generations of some blissful ignorance about where food comes from, and how to keep children healthy. These both fell more under the domain of mothers in the first half of the twentieth century than they do now, but both have been deferred to the food and pharmaceutical industries by most of us today. A visit to the local dairy to *see* where some of our food came from was de rigueur in my elementary school, as was a lesson in how to churn butter in my kindergarten. That was in 1965 (it sounds like 1865), but teachings such as these have long fallen away. With the introduction of high-fructose corn syrup into many processed foods in the 1980s, an absolute explosion of products made just for children tumbled onto supermarket shelves and kitchen cupboards, from purple cereal and Day-Glo orange drinks to pink yogurt and rainbow sprinkled frosting. When I first began my private practice in 1999, I was stunned to realize that many moms did not have the foggiest notion about how to prepare food. They did not grow up cooking, never learned to do it in school, nor did they see their parents do much cooking—though they had seen a lot of microwaving! We haven't thought too much about what's really in things such as tomatoes, chickens, or fast-food French fries, nor have we questioned much about what's in the medications we've been advised to give our children.

As our children have literally become more chronically ill and disabled than ever before, it seems that moment has passed.

There is an urgency felt among many parents to turn this around, to swap in as many good things as we can, to rear healthy kids. Good food is definitely one of those things. In whatever way possible, teach your children about cooking and eating healthy food together, even if it is only rarely possible. What's healthy? Many parents I meet are worried that this means making their kids strictly avoid parties, fats, every artificial color, and eating mostly vegetables, fruit, raw foods, or salads. Not exactly. Healthy can mean roasting a locally raised chicken yourself instead of buying one injected with mysterious flavorings, and serving it with homemade mashed potatoes—not spuds from instant flakes, but from actual potatoes—maybe even organic ones. It can mean baking a gluten-free pumpkin bread with coconut milk and ghee in it, instead of wheat flour, cow's milk, and butter, because your child is gluten- and dairy-intolerant. This is a sweet and indulgent treat, but at least you're not buying a supermarket doughnut or muffin made with trans fats, corn syrup, and proteins they react to. It can mean gluten-free crepes for breakfast, filled with fresh strawberries and drizzled with a little dark chocolate (not as hard or time-consuming as you might think). Though this will seem like a fancy dessert to a child, it actually gives good start-of-day calories, a smidge of fiber, potassium, vitamins A and C in the fruit, and some protein from the eggs in the crepe batter. It can mean planting lettuce this summer, or some peas or carrots—some of the easiest-to-grow items around—to pique your children's interest in what that stuff tastes like when it comes from their own backyard. Or maybe it's easiest for you to spring for a juicing machine, and let your children try putting anything and everything (fruit and vegetable, that is) into it, to see what concoctions they like best. They might be very surprised to see how good it tastes to *drink* a fresh organic apple, with a stalk or two of celery and a carrot, spun together in a juicer. Avail yourself of the virtually unlimited resources on the Internet for finding recipes, trying a kitchen garden, getting a school garden going, or using a community garden plot. No one needs to be a superhero about this. Robyn O'Brien, author of *Unhealthy Truth*, coined the "80/20" rule to encourage parents to focus on getting good food in the picture, most of the time: If you can do this 80 percent of the time, don't sweat the other 20 percent—that is, let go of those times when kids may eat the fluffy pink cupcake at a friend's birthday party. There are many small and simple ways to engage a love of good, healthful eating in your home, and your children will be better off for it.

The other part of the equation for nutrition-focused tools is using supplements. Whether or not a child should add supplements depends on his or her individual needs, and this is what I assess for families in my practice. Supplement strategies can quickly feel overwhelming. Check with your naturopath or pediatrician on the items you choose, or let them choose some for you. Once you get to choosing which ones to use, a few tips are helpful, so you can feel confident that you are not wasting your money. As for safety, supplements have a good record. Obvious precautions: If you are not certain about the safety of any supplement (or medication, for that matter), don't use it. Seek out professional guidance. A prime example: Iron supplements are poisonous when used incorrectly. Don't give your child any supplemental iron without running it by your pediatrician first. A daily chewable multivitamin is fine for ordinary circumstances in kids—but because these usually contain iron and taste good to kids, they may gobble several if allowed. Don't let this happen. Keep these out of your child's reach, to prevent poisoning from the iron in them.

Dietary Supplement Standards

The FDA is responsible for monitoring dietary supplements. Recently, this agency established good manufacturing practices (GMP), which supplement makers are required to follow. But just as has been true with identifying problematic foods—such as spinach that contains salmonella or ground beef that is contaminated with *E. coli*—the FDA is overwhelmed, and not able to keep up with the infinite demands of monitoring our food, drugs, or supplements. At the very least, a supplement should carry a GMP seal. GMP aims to ensure that supplements have what they say they have in them for ingredients, and nothing else, in the amounts specified. It also aims to eliminate contaminants, which can occur in everything, from foods to medicines and vaccines to supplements.

GMP is a step in the right direction, but many manufacturers are interested in a higher standard. A voluntary quality standard that some manufacturers self-impose is the "USP Voluntary Dietary Supplement Program." "USP" is the United States Pharmacopeia, which is a nongovernmental, standards-setting authority for dietary supplements, prescription and over-the-counter medicines, and other health care products manufactured or sold in the United States. USP standards for food ingredients and dietary supplements are widely recognized, and the USP itself has a long history—it first convened in 1820 to set quality standards for medications, and has worked with government, industry, and health care providers ever since. USP standards go beyond GMP by requiring on-site visits by volunteer expert inspectors, and by requiring proof that a supplement breaks down, releases, and delivers its contents as intended. There are more than a thousand volunteer experts working with USP, under strict conflict-of-interest codes that are arguably stronger than the FDA's. A good supplement will carry the USP mark. You can learn more about this at USP.org.

Still other dietary supplement manufacturers will prefer to make their products available through only licensed health care providers, in order to control how they are used and ensure they will be used effectively and safely. These are usually more expensive than store brands because these manufacturers often impose even higher quality standards. One example of this is a TGA certificate, issued by the Therapeutic Goods Association of Australia, considered one of the most stringent standards worldwide. It requires regular on-site auditing as well. Some manufacturers impose their own standards for in-house or independently monitored quality control, and this is what you are usually buying when you buy products that cost more.

Can You Trust Providers Who Sell Stuff?

Many providers working with nutrition-focused tools sell supplements. This is often a bone of contention with naysayers in the medical community, who claim that the only reason a provider would sell supplements is to fleece innocent health consumers. While there are always unscrupulous individuals, on balance, most health professionals take their training and ethics seriously. Many parents don't realize that pediatricians "sell stuff," too, in that they earn significant revenues from vaccinations, including bonuses and grants when quotas are met.* Both types of providers fervently believe in the products they are selling, whether it's you or your health insurance company doing the buying, and both will cite science to back their beliefs. It's overly simple to say that supplements don't help anyone. Of course they do—like medications, when used correctly, they can be very effective. The important piece is establishing trust with your providers, so that if you (or your insurance plan) are buying products through them, you feel confident and positive about it. If a product obtained through a provider has not helped your child, whether it's a medication, a vaccine, or a supplement, be sure to say so, so that you can work together on healthier, more effective options.

In my own practice, I have avoided selling supplements for the most part. With two or three exceptions that I've made for truly unique products, I prefer to let my clients comparison shop for items I recommend, which is easy to do online. I recommend many different manufacturers' products, depending on the child's needs, the product formulation, and the product's format (liquid, chewable, gel, topical, or medical food). It would be a challenge for me to maintain a stock of the varied items I would need in a supplement pharmacy, and I would rather remain unbiased about this anyway, by not selling these items myself. I also have not found that a single manufacturer makes a product line capable of

---

* See "Do Doctors Have a Financial Incentive to Get Their Patients Fully Vaccinated?" on AskDrSears.com, and "The Impact of Physician Bonuses, Enhanced Fees, and Feedback on Childhood Immunization Coverage Rates" in the *American Journal of Public Health* (February 1999) for more information.

meeting the diverse needs of all the children I encounter, and would likely have to carry inventory from at least six manufacturers to attempt this. If your provider is recommending that you buy a product in his office, feel free to make the purchase or say no, if you'd like to search online for better pricing. Consider that shipping fees will be tacked onto your Internet purchase. You should use exactly what your provider has recommended, and not a substitute. Even items sold only by providers are often available (at discounted prices) online, much to the dismay of both the manufacturer and the provider, who would rather see these tools used with closer monitoring. You can also ask your provider why a product he is selling is advantageous or necessary, over and above what you might pick up at a big-box drugstore or supermarket.

Dietary supplements definitely vary in quality and efficacy, depending on how they are manufactured, formulated, stored, and administered. Resources abound on the web that review supplements, to help you answer this question. One site called Consumer Labs.com offers an online subscription service that provides reviews of supplement quality and safety. Another, SupplementQuality.com, offers free information about dietary supplement standards and regulations, what to look for in individual supplements, what different quality seals mean, and what questions you should ask a manufacturer, to vet the quality, efficacy, and safety of a product. Another interesting site, NutraIngredients-USA.com, monitors the supplement industry, and you can catch up on regulatory news, press releases on scientific studies relating to supplements, and new product innovations. You can also visit the FDA's website to learn about supplement quality control. Some are especially worth the higher price, while for others, premium pricing is less important.

Where to Splurge: Fish Oils, Omega-3 Fatty Acids, and Probiotics

A few supplements aren't worth buying cheaply. Fish oils are one of them. Omega-3 fatty acids in fish oils continue to show more and more promise for modulating inflammation in all kinds of conditions, from heart and vascular diseases to rheumatoid arthritis to asthma and allergies. Their role in mood disorders, cognition, and activating areas of the brain responsible for executive function is impressive as well. Before using fish oils for those wonderful omega-3 fatty acids, be sure that fish is not an inflammatory food for your child. Some kids in my caseload are anaphylactic to all kinds of fish, and have to use other sources. One child I encountered with asthma was being given fish oils to get the anti-inflammatory benefits, only to find that he was reactive to it on an IgE panel! Fish also concentrate human-sourced toxins from our oceans into their own livers and fatty tissues, so the older and bigger the fish, the more toxin-laden it will be. Reputable manufacturers of fish oil supplements will follow strict methods to keep mercury, other heavy metals, PCBs, or other contaminants out of their products. If it's safe for your child to have fish, these oils can be great, and they come in everything from chewable gummy candies to orange-flavored gel caps that burst when chewed, to pudding-like gels that squirt on foods or on the tongue, to liquids and large capsules to swallow. Rules of thumb for fish oils are:

- Check that the manufacturer screens its product for heavy metal content, since these accumulate in cod liver and fish oils, as do polychlorinated biphenyls (PCBs). Though a test by *Consumer Reports* didn't find detectable levels of these in any fish oil products tested, still use a product from a company committed to imposing strict standards in this regard. Examples would be Nordic Naturals or Pharmax.

- Check potency. Cheaper brands of fish oils usually deliver less DHA and EPA per dose. They often supply half the amount of these fatty acids than more expensive brands, meaning you will need to use twice the amount to get a relevant dose—thereby eradicating the savings you think you may be getting. Children can use between 1 and 4 grams of combined DHA and EPA daily. Some products supply only 50 milligrams per dose, which is not nearly enough to produce much benefit, per research that has accumulated so far.

- Buy it refrigerated, and keep it that way. Fish oils are highly susceptible to rancidity, as anyone knows who has bought or cooked fish. Fish oil supplements in any form should be refrigerated once they are opened. Though it may not be deemed necessary by the manufacturer, keep fish oil capsules refrigerated, too. Rancid fish oils will smell and taste bad. This means that they are full of free oxygen radical species that can do harm to cell chemistry. Don't use rancid fish oil.

- Consider brands that use processing that best preserves the native state of the fish oils, so the oils in them are easiest to digest and absorb as intended.

- For chewables and gels, make sure that the additional ingredients in the capsule or gel itself aren't contraindicated for your child. For example, some manufacturers will use soy oil to make gels or as a filler ingredient in the capsule; others commonly use citrus for flavor, which is inflammatory for some children. One brand of fish oil, Coromega gel, is a hit with kids because of its texture and flavor. It's easy to squirt on waffles, pancakes, or even cupcakes. But this product contains egg, so will be contraindicated for those with egg allergy.

Probiotics are another product not to skimp on, if you are going to spend on them at all. Cheap probiotics usually come with filler ingredients that have no (or dubious) therapeutic benefit. They will also not tell you how many colony forming units (CFUs) are delivered per dose, and may only say that a dose has something like 500 milligrams of live cultures. Skip it. Better probiotic manufacturers guarantee the viability and potency of their product through its expiration date. The label will say that a dose delivers a certain number of guaranteed live colony–forming units, not a vague assertion of a volume or weight of powder—and that number should be high—that is, well into the billions per dose. A reasonable starting dose of a probiotic for a child is 8 billion CFUs per day, and even this is too low for many circumstances. Some products, such as Culturelle, deliver a single strain of beneficial bacteria, while others, such as Udo's Choice, deliver multiple strains. What is right for your child can be best ascertained by a provider experienced in using these, but if you are trying them on your own, look for products that guarantee high potency in explicit terms. If probiotic supplements don't improve GI symptoms such as diarrhea or constipation within about four weeks, it's likely that a different product is needed—either the same strains in higher potency, different strains altogether, or a strong antimicrobial herb or prescription may be needed to address a bowel infection that probiotics alone can't remedy.

You can also buy probiotics from your provider's office. Manufacturers such as Klaire Labs and Pharmax make probiotics to sell through providers only, for example. Different probiotic blends have different applications, and your naturopath or gastroenterologist are good experts to ask. One popular strain is *Saccharomyces boulardii*; this is actually a strain of *yeast* that doesn't particularly like to colonize a human gut, but it will go to work to eradicate unwanted flora for you. Clinical reviews have repeatedly shown it to be effective in reducing *Clostridia difficile* bacteria in the intestine, a microbe that can trigger chronic diarrhea and malabsorption. It can be combined with antibiotics to help keep your child's bowel flora in balance, if an antibiotic is needed. A caution with *S. boulardii*: Avoid using it beyond 30 days, as it may become too entrenched in the gut, and trigger symptoms of yeast overgrowth.

If probiotics don't seem confusing enough, there are also "prebiotics" to consider. These are available as a separate supplement, together with the probiotic, or even in some foods. *Prebiotics* aren't live bacteria cultures. They are food for the bacterial cultures. Specifically, they are certain types of carbohydrates that beneficial bacterial species like to eat. You may have seen "fructooligosaccharide (FOS)" on a food or supplement label. This is a prebiotic; it is a carbohydrate food source for the beneficial bacteria. Others are lactulose, galactooligosaccharides, or inulin. Still more exist, and need further study. More research has been done on using prebiotics in infants than adults, and it appears that these can benefit healthy colonization of a baby's gut, especially if the baby is formula fed and not breast-fed. Prebiotics are added to some infant formulas, and are becoming popular ingredients in juices, drinks, and smoothies. Infants and children struggling with inflammation, necrotizing enterocolitis, or eosinophilic esophagitis should be working with their providers on effective protocols to supplement prebiotics and probiotics. Cautions for prebiotics are simple: Too much will cause a lot of gas, bloating, or loose stool. It's best to start with a low dose if you use these, increase slowly, and stop if it triggers spikes in physical symptoms or behavior. In children who do not digest carbohydrates and starches very well, prebiotics can be especially poorly tolerated, and parents often report sudden aggressive or reactive behavior as the only symptom. In this case, the prebiotic may be usurped by undesirable bowel flora instead; this will trigger a spike in organic acids excreted by those flora, which in turn are absorbed systemically and appear to have behavioral effects. This is why kids on the Specific Carbohydrate Diet usually should avoid prebiotics, because they are larger than allowed carbohydrate molecules for that diet. Until I am certain that carbohydrates are well tolerated in a child, I usually defer prebiotics. I also avoid products that add glutamine to the probiotic blend, since glutamine can be poorly tolerated by children with autism, with mood disorders and mood swings, seizures, or difficulty with modulating behavior or aggression.

Expect to hear more about probiotics as medical research catches up with the trends on this. Our understanding of these microbes as critical modulators of immune response is just beginning, both early in life and as we age. This is a key piece for children with special needs. For prevention of certain cancers, mitigating allergies and asthma, and just helping us have comfortable bowel habits daily, beneficial microflora have been too long overlooked for their contribution.

Daily Multi

It pays to be choosy about multivitamins for kids, but this doesn't mean you must spend forty or fifty dollars on the right item. In some cases, children need very specific protocols for replenishing full complements of micronutrients. In this scenario, work with a knowledgeable provider. If you simply need a basic daily insurance policy for vitamins and minerals, a multivitamin can be a great help without being costly. Multivitamins for children are cheaper when they are low potency and use inexpensive fillers and flavors. An example of this is your garden-variety chewable tablets or drops that give a little bit of vitamins A, C, and D, some of the B vitamins, maybe a smidge of zinc, and perhaps a dot of iron. These are fine for kids in good health who have no special needs and who have no issues for nutritional depletion or malabsorption. That pretty much excludes all the kids in my caseload, who do have something or other going on nutritionally, and need higher potencies of vitamins and minerals to overcome these issues. Whether it's a poor total intake, lots of inflammation, chronic diarrhea or constipation, or a rigid eating pattern, the kids I meet tend to be drained of some essential nutrients.

I often recommend larger than usual nutrient doses for a specific purpose, such as using higher doses of B vitamins alongside tyrosine, to help slow movers get going in the morning and be able to focus a bit more at school, or using iron judiciously to treat anemia, chromium to bracket blood sugar swings, or zinc to repair the depletion of this mineral that is common for kids who eat a lot of yogurt, milk, cheese, and wheat foods. Most store-bought brands of children's multivitamins are low potency, and low value for kids with high special needs. They tend to overlook adequate essential minerals by giving inadequate doses of zinc (3–10 milligrams), difficult-to-absorb iron (ferrous sulfate), and no selenium, iodine, chromium, or magnesium. They also usually include copper, which is frequently avoided in some circumstances in children with special needs (autism, psychiatric conditions, or high inflammation). You can work with a provider to choose multis for your child that don't break the bank, but do a much better job for special situations, such as ProThera Vita-Tab chewables, Klaire Labs Vita Spectrum powder or capsules, Rainbow Light NutriStars, Metagenics Chewable, or Kirkman Children's Chewables. There are also liquid suspensions from manufacturers such as Pharmax, Metagenics, and many others that work well for kids. Look for a product that gives minerals as well as vitamins, not just vitamins alone.

While it isn't appropriate to give children adult multivitamins or supplements, or to necessarily give 100 percent or more of the recommended amount of every nutrient in a multi, it is notable that higher than government recommended levels of supplements are often given to children by providers using nutrition-focused tools. This is because, once again, we are talking about children with heightened health needs of all sorts. Recommended levels on labels of dietary supplements for children are based on data sets of well, neurotypical children with no health concerns. Chronic conditions, acute illnesses, and infections change how nutrients are used, and how much of them we may need. The government has made no attempt to state how much of any nutrient anyone needs in special circumstances such as these. This is why it is helpful to get input from a provider familiar with current research on nutrition in pediatric special-needs circumstances, when you are considering supplements for your child.

For essential minerals—iron, zinc, chromium, selenium, calcium, molybdenum, iodine, and magnesium—many brands are available, and you can shop for good pricing. Mineral supplements should be held to high standards for purity and for being free of heavy metal contaminants. B-group vitamins and vitamin C generally have lower toxicity because they are water soluble and easily excreted if we have more than we need. But minerals are stored in tissues, so they must be used in the correct dose to avoid toxic effects, in the right form, and at times when they are best absorbed relative to meals, foods, other supplements, or medications. Minerals occur in many different forms in foods and supplements, and vary for how easily they are absorbed. Medications can interfere with their absorption, increase their absorption, synergize their effects, and vice versa. A great resource on this is your local pharmacist. Ask about drug-nutrient interactions before you add supplements to your child's regimen. Different forms can be useful for specific purposes. For example, if a child needs calming magnesium but has constipation, I may choose magnesium citrate as the supplemental form. If a child has loose stools, then I may choose magnesium glycinate, which is less laxative. Calcium carbonate is the form in most children's calcium supplements, but it may not be wise for a child who needs to avoid high-oxalate foods. In this scenario, calcium citrate with meals is often suggested instead. Like most minerals, zinc is also available in several forms: zinc sulfate, picolinate, gluconate, citrate, acetate, glycinate, or monomethionine; of these, research favors the glycinate form as easiest to absorb and most effective at raising serum zinc level, reducing oxidative stress, and for fabricating a protein called metallothionein, which we need to remove toxic heavy metals from the body. This is yet another example of how cheaper is not necessarily better; much more of the cheaper stuff, zinc sulfate, would be needed to do the same job.

Zinc competes with copper, iron, magnesium, and calcium for absorption. If your child needs to use a separate high dose of zinc, such as a 30-milligram capsule of zinc picolinate, it is best taken with some food for best assimilation and least stomach upset. Chromium has become controversial because of a study that tested the effects of extremely high doses of chromium picolinate on hamster cell cultures. The tissue cultures developed genetic damage consistent with cancer. Critics point out that the doses used were astronomically higher than what is in supplements, and that administering the doses to tissue cultures is not analogous to oral ingestion. Later studies exonerated chromium picolonate enough to prompt the CDC to declare that it is a safe supplement, leaving many with diabetes relieved, as it is often used to improve blood glucose control. Children can use it for this purpose, too, but should not use doses far above the daily recommended intake (15–25 micrograms, not milligrams) for long periods of time without professional guidance. Children using medications to control blood sugar should know that taking chromium may synergize the medication; discuss how this affects your child's medication dose with your doctor.

What about just B vitamins alone? Adding B vitamin complex supplements for children is safe to do—excess amounts of these will simply wash out daily in urine. But will this do your child any good? This is where your health care provider needs to step up. If you would like to try some of these, the caveats to know are:

- Extrasensitive children (those who seem to react to all kinds of foods, additives, or inhaled allergens) sometimes get exceedingly hyper or irritable on large doses of B-group vitamins.

- Others with untreated intestinal candida overgrowth or other microbial infections in the gut may overreact in this way, too. "Gut bugs" love B vitamins!

- Don't give B vitamins at bedtime, as they tend to make us more alert, wakeful, or energetic rather than calm.

- Start with ordinary doses that fall at or just above the recommended dietary reference intake (DRI). B vitamins are available at many thousands of times above the DRI. While this may be beneficial in some instances, it can also trigger irritability or hyperactivity.

- Vitamin B6 is pyridoxine. The active form of this in cells is called pyridoxal-5-phosphate (P5P). Some products contain both forms, which may be too activating for your child. Ask your provider for guidance.

- In the United States, many foods containing wheat are fortified with B vitamins, while foods made with gluten-free grains are not. So when children are on gluten-free diets, it is especially important that they either eat foods that supply B vitamins or that they use a supplement with full DRIs for the B-group daily. Foods that deliver the B-group include turkey, lentils, bananas, melons, potatoes, nuts, salmon, eggs, and tempeh.

Unlike B vitamins, which quickly exit in urine if they are not needed and have very low toxicity, vitamin A is fat soluble and can thus build up in tissues such as the liver. Avoid too much of a good thing with vitamin A. This is available at high doses in many specialty multivitamins marketed to the autism community. A teaspoon of cod liver oil also delivers a good dose, more than smaller children would need in a day. Too much is toxic, and can trigger pain (especially headaches or pain in shins), poor appetite, hair loss, and skin changes. I have encountered children with vitamin A toxicity, usually from cod liver oil or high-dose supplements that were used for too long. It can make children irritable and agitated, too. If your child has used more than 4000 international units of vitamin A daily for months, and you note any of these signs, you can ask your doctor to check vitamin A status with a blood test. You may need to withdraw vitamin A for several weeks to allow levels to normalize.

Vitamin D is also fat soluble, but it is much harder to reach an excessive dose. Up until recently, only a few hundred international units of vitamin D were recommended daily for adults and children. As study after study rolls in on the importance of this vitamin, it's clear that we need much more than previously thought. Individuals who are dark skinned don't make as much of it with sun exposure as fair-skinned persons. Vitamin D levels were lowest in persons with autism and schizophrenia, in a study that scrutinized over one hundred adults with psychiatric diagnoses; their diagnostic presentations improved with Vitamin D replenishment. It is a more potent immune modulator than we have appreciated, and has been shown to mitigate autoimmune responses—which has enormous implications for conditions such as diabetes, celiac disease, autism, allergies, cancer, and cystic fibrosis.

How much vitamin D should kids with special needs use? Recommendations for typical, healthy children have been bumped up into the range of 1000–5000 international units, depending on age and weight. Is there a place for very high doses to be used therapeutically? It probably won't be long before researchers look at that. So far, I am aware of two anecdotes of children given tens of thousands of international units of vitamin D daily for several weeks by mistake; there are surely many more. One had autism, and one had Down's syndrome. Neither child was injured; neither had toxic effects. Both children started talking a lot more, and showed new alertness and cognitive ability. Both had initiated vitamin D supplementation when their doctors found subpar vitamin D levels with a blood test. In each case, the doctors gave the mothers instructions to replenish vitamin D but with a much lower dose. The moms in these anecdotes both gave dropperfuls, instead of a single drop or two, of vitamin D daily. One child was given 150,000 international units daily for six weeks. The other received 25,000 international units daily for three weeks. Both had dramatic improvements using these doses, but stopped once the error was discovered. Exactly how this nutrient should be used and what it may do for special-needs kids remains to be seen. At the very least, give 1000 international units to infants and toddlers, 3000 international units to school-age children, and as much as 5000 international units to high school kids daily, as vitamin D3 drops, and stay tuned to research around this so you can discuss it with your doctor or naturopath.

Many other supplement tools—hundreds of them—exist both for nutrients known and established as critical for life, and for other compounds that may have functional benefits, such as coenzyme Q10, alpha lipoic acid, N-acetyl cysteine, and so on. Reviewing and understanding them all can't fit here. Use this chapter as a guide for some safe and essential baseline supplement tools your child can use. For more detail, along with talking to your providers, look into books such as *Prescription for Nutritional Healing*. This is an encyclopedic reference of hundreds of nutrients, supplements, and herbs that can support your efforts in using nutrition-focused tools.

Books, Links, and Tips

Here are some resources that can support you in exploring pharm-free health maintenance tools for your family. Stepping off the pharmaceutical merry-go-round for our children's health care needs can be hard. Medications are tightly intertwined into our pediatric care delivery system, and training in other options is sparse for our physicians. So you may not hear much about other paths at your pediatrician's office. When I was expecting my son in 1996, the books of choice for new moms were the What to Expect series—but these didn't do me much good. The advice was too generic for my circumstances, and when the text did approach some of the challenges I faced, the advice fell short, often ending with an "ask your doctor" mantra that quickly wore out for me. In our case, the doctor usually *didn't* have answers or strategies that worked, and it wasn't long before I realized many other young families were having the same experience. This is what ultimately led me to do the work I do today, and to write books for parents like me. Here are some wonderful books that I wish I'd had back then. I discovered some of them early in my parenting journey and found that they indeed helped create the health and wellness my baby deserved. Others came along a little later, and I still encounter books today to add to my library of the many wonderful titles for families who are compelled to reach beyond the scope of conventional Western medical practice. Here are some of my favorites:

Books for Integrative Pediatrics

Cave, Stephanie, MD, FAAFP, *What Your Doctor May Not Tell You About Childhood Immunizations* (2001, 2010).

Cummings, Stephen, MD, and Dana Ullman, MPH, *Everybody's Guide to Homeopathic Medicines* (3rd revised edition, 2004).

Feder, Lauren, MD, *Natural Baby and Childcare: Practical Medical Advice and Holistic Wisdom for Raising Healthy Children* (2006).

Lansky, Amy, PhD, *Impossible Cure: The Promise of Homeopathy* (2003).

Lydall, Wendy, *Raising a Vaccine Free Child* (2009).

Murphy, Jamie, *What Every Parent Should Know About Childhood Immunizations* (1993).

O'Brien, Robyn, *Unhealthy Truth* (2009).

Reichenberg-Ullman, Judyth, and Robert Ullman, *Prozac-Free: Homeopathic Medicine for Depression, Anxiety, and Other Mental and Emotional Problems* (1999).

Reichenberg-Ullman, Judyth, and Robert Ullman, *Ritalin-Free Kids: Safe and Effective Homeopathic Medicine for ADD and Other Behavioral and Learning Problems* (1996).

Reichenberg-Ullman, Judyth, Robert Ullman, Ian Luepker, and Bernard Rimland, *A Drug-Free Approach to Asperger Syndrome and Autism: Homeopathic Care for Exceptional Kids* (2005).

Sears, Robert, MD, FAAP, *The Vaccine Book: Making the Right Decision for Your Child* (2007).

Here are some of the many websites supporting families on the complementary medicine or integrative pediatrics path:

American Personal Rights
AmericanPersonalRights.org

Healthy Homeopathy
HealthyHomeopathy.com

Holistic Moms Network
HolisticMoms.org

Life Health Choices
LifeHealthChoices.com

Mothering Magazine
Mothering.com

Natural News
NaturalNews.com

Organic Consumers Association
OrganicConsumers.org

Parental Rights
ParentalRights.org

Weston Price Foundation
WestonAPrice.org

Special Needs Advocacy

Protect your child's right to free and appropriate education (FAPE) by getting informed on education law. School districts nationwide are squeezed to accommodate more children with special needs than ever, with less federal funding—the percentage of federal contributions to programs mandated under the Individuals with Disabilities Education Act was substantially cut in 2005. Unfortunately, this means children do get left behind, as districts scramble to save money—especially children with special needs, who cost about twice as much per pupil to educate than typical peers. This also means parents must become sturdy advocates for their children's right to access education that is appropriate. It is cheaper for schools to group special-needs children into segregated classrooms away from typical peers, but not necessarily legal or appropriate. Parents who simply agree to whatever a school district dictates are possibly waiving many of their children's rights without knowing it. WrightsLaw.com is a "sped" advocacy site rich with tools and information about legal precedents, case law in education, and special needs. Other helpful sites abound; check out SPRLaw.net and SpecialEdLaw .blogs.com.

Cookbooks for Special Diets

As hard as it is to change how you run your kitchen or organize meals for your family, if it will make your child healthier, do it. Be encouraged to know that this is much easier now that it was ten years ago. Besides an Internet now overflowing with recipes that are just a click away, there are more cookbooks and specialized foods than ever before. Eating food that's organic, allergen-free, additive-free, or less processed costs more at the grocery checkout, but can pay off in health visits you won't be making for infections, illness, cavities, or other health problems. For strategies on transitioning to special diets, how to succeed with these for your child, plus a few recipes, see my previous book, *Special-Needs Kids Eat Right*, published in 2009.

Capone, Mary, *The Gluten-Free Italian Cookbook: Classic Cuisine from the Italian Countryside* (2008). This book is beautiful to look at and easy to read. Its forte is that author Mary Capone is a celiac who has the good fortune of a true Italian heritage with many "kitchen angels," as she calls them—loving relatives who handed down their culinary secrets. It has everything Italian in it—from wedding soup to homemade tortellini to tiramisu—all gluten-free. Suggestions for accommodating a dairy-free version are often included in her recipes. Both ambitious and easy recipes are included: A simple one for breakfast popovers can be made in minutes, filled with fruit, jam, butter, scrambled eggs, or even chocolate, if you are really splurging.

Reilly, Rebecca, *Gluten-Free Baking* (2002). This is a favorite I've mentioned before. Before I found this book, my efforts to include my son in the usual treats for special occasions were tolerated more than celebrated. Gluten-free pie crusts, cakes, cookies, sweet breads, and more were demystified for me with this book, authored by a trained pasty chef whose daughter turned out to be gluten-intolerant.

Segerten, Alissa, and Tom Malterre, MS, CN, *Whole Life Nutrition Cookbook: Whole Foods Recipes for Personal and Planetary Health* (2nd edition, 2009). This is both a cookbook and an instructional resource for information on special diets and whole foods, all in one book. It includes more than two hundred recipes that are gluten-, dairy-, and egg-free.

Specialized Formulas

When children have allergy, sensitivity, or intolerance to more than a few foods, it can become literally impossible to give them enough to eat. If you are avoiding more than four or five major proteins for your child, chances are (according to research on children with food allergies) your child is not growing as well as expected, and does not eat as many nutrients and calories as peers without allergies. As I've discussed in this book and in *Special-Needs Kids Eat Right*, whether or not this is true in your child's case can be assessed with a nutrition consult by a licensed nutrition professional or registered dietitian. Your pediatrician will probably not analyze a food diary for you, which is just one part of what needs to be reviewed when growth patterns falter. He also probably won't calculate the per-pound nutrient needs for your child either, because he is not trained to do that. But this is helpful and necessary, when children are facing surgery for insertion of a gastrostomy tube. Before moving to that invasive option, you may be able to see your child rebound with specialized formulas used correctly as an oral feed.

Growth patterns will reliably recover when children are given the right amounts—and *types*—of calories. They have to be able to absorb these normally, too. In some cases, it's clear a child can't attain a food intake that will correct her growth pattern, either because a diet is too restrictive, because of a self-imposed picky eating pattern, or because of delayed oral motor skills. Once children reach a certain low in their growth pattern, their calorie needs per pound can double or even triple. Even in normal growth status, children need about twice the calories per pound that adults do. To put this in perspective, a toddler in growth failure might need a calorie intake that would be akin to an adult eating over 10,000 calories every day, for weeks.

This is a scenario that warrants specialized formulas. It simply isn't possible to put all that bulk into a small child, without resorting to calorie-dense medical foods. The upside of these is that they usually work very well. The downside is that because they are not real food, but conglomerations of individual nutrients, many parents object to using them out of concern that they are "artificial." They are indeed artificially concocted, with easy-to-tolerate, nonallergenic sources of fats, carbohydrates, and protein; they provide nutrients in forms that a normally functioning intestine liberates from whole food. Children needing them are, for various reasons, unable to extract nutrients out of food very well, or can't absorb them without inflammation. These formulas bypass that, and provide the nutrients in their most accessible format.

The most common complaint about these formulas is that children refuse them—they don't like the taste. A motivating factor for families is understanding that if a child needing this tool refuses it as an oral feeding, the next step is likely to be feeding the exact same stuff in a tube. Manufacturers make their best effort at flavoring these with the least offensive ingredients. SHS North America, makers of Neocate and Splash, have pledged to use non-GMO maltodextrin sourced from corn in some of their products, and have removed aspartame (NutraSweet). Others attempt a more natural presentation for their product, such as Ultracare for Kids from Metagenics.

So far, in my opinion, no one has quite figured it out—there is no such thing as natural or organic medical food, because once again, these are not real food, not natural, and they must be artificially formulated. But I look forward to the day when manufacturers formulate something a bit more palatable with fewer artificial flavors for these children. In any case, I encourage parents to try these when warranted. They are most effective when used with professional guidance. You can inquire about insurance coverage for these as well. Your allergist, gastroenterologist, or pediatrician will likely have to go to bat for you in order to access insurance coverage for these formulas. Some states only reim-

burse them when used in tube feedings; states with more pro-
gressive insurance mandates *require* coverage for these formulas
for oral feeding, under certain nutrition diagnoses. States that
have nutrition care mandates that may cover these formulas for
oral feeding are Arizona, Connecticut, Illinois, Maine, Maryland,
Massachusetts, Minnesota, New Hampshire, New Jersey, New
York, Rhode Island, and Texas. Be sure to check with your GI specialist or allergist team, to learn about other products that may not
be mentioned here.

**Neocate Infant, Neocate Junior, Neocate One Plus (all powdered)
and Splash (ready to drink in a "juice box" format).** These are amino
acid–based (elemental) formulas that provide complete nutrition
for children with gastrointestinal impairment. I have successfully
used these products for over a decade, for kids with autism,
growth failure, and multiple food protein intolerance or allergy.
Note: Corn syrup solids, corn-sourced maltodextrin, or corn syrup
are used as the carbohydrate source in these, because it is gluten-
free, and because it helps kids accept the taste. There is no cross-
contamination with corn protein. Some children will tolerate this
carbohydrate source poorly if they have untreated bowel infections or enzyme insufficiencies for digesting carbs. Visit Neocate
.com for details. You can also get insurance coding information for
these formulas at the Neocate site or at NutritionCare.net.

Elecare. This is also an amino acid–based formula for children
over one year, but it is available only as a powder to reconstitute.
One advantage Elecare has over the Neocate and Splash products
is that it is available in a vanilla flavor, while Neocate and Splash
are available only in "tropical," orange-pineapple, lemon, grape,
and a chocolate that isn't quite chocolately. Some children will
prefer the vanilla flavor.

Nutramigen and Alimentum for infants; Peptamen Junior and Pepdite for children over one year. These are semi-elemental formulas, meaning that the protein source in them starts with an actual food protein such as casein or soy, and is enzymatically treated to be partly digested. This leaves smaller peptides that are easier to digest. Some children with food allergy or GI impairment can tolerate these, but in my experience, many children cannot. If you have a child with autism, these formulas would be contraindicated on a gluten-free, casein-free diet. The one exception here may be Pepdite, which uses hydrolyzed (enzymatically treated) soy protein as a protein source. Some children have managed well with this in my caseload. Each product mentioned here has consumer support websites and hotlines where you can get more information about trying them. Your pediatrician may not know much about these, but a pediatric gastroenterologist or registered dietitian will.

Utracare for Kids. This is a medical food from the functional medicine supplement company Metagenics. It is a powder with 120 calories per scoop that can be mixed with water, juice, or whatever your child likes. The protein source is rice—a poor source that Metagenics augments with the amino acids lysine, threonine, and taurine to improve its nutritional value. Vitamins and minerals are added also. This formula has 250 milligrams of calcium per scoop as well, which limits how much a child should consume in a day to two to four scoops, depending on how much calcium he receives from other foods and supplements. Some children prefer this product's vanilla flavor, but it is not a complete nutrition source as the formulas mentioned above are. It also has a sandy texture, which some kids reject. It should not be used as an infant formula.

Modular tools. "Modular" means patching a formula out of individual ingredients, and this is something I often do in practice. When I need a high-value protein source—equivalent to what would be found in an egg or meat—but can't use those foods in a child's diet for various reasons, I create modular feeding options for children, based on their calculated needs for protein, calories, fats, and carbs daily. It may also be true that the products I've mentioned already don't work. In those cases, modular tools can work well. To do this, I employ a free amino acid, complete protein source such as SHS North America Essential Amino Acid Mix (see SHSNA.com) or my own formulation, Learn Grow Thrive Amino Action (see NutritionCare.net). These are blends of essential amino acids, which are what dietary protein yields when digestion is working normally and when food proteins trigger no inflammation. Therapeutically, they are used in ordinary doses—that is, in amounts that might be found in a glass of milk or a typical meal with protein foods—two or three times per day. They can be stirred into cold or warm soft foods, or mixed into smoothies and shakes. They don't dissolve well in plain juices or milk substitutes, without some other ingredients to distract from their appearance or taste.

An example of a modular option recipe:

½ cup or large scoop So Delicious brand coconut-based chocolate or vanilla "ice cream" (gluten-, casein-, and soy-free)

1 teaspoon Learn Grow Thrive Amino Action (about 5 grams total protein)

½ teaspoon agave syrup

dash gluten-free vanilla

4 ounces vanilla-flavored almond milk

½ teaspoon flax oil

½ teaspoon safflower oil

This can be modified to use fruit, any milk substitute, vanilla "ice cream," medium chain triglycerides (an easy-to-absorb fat source), carrot juice, or whatever your child likes. It can also be formulated to deliver a lower oxalate load by using certain fruits, vanilla "ice cream," and coconut or rice milk instead of nut milk and chocolate-flavored "ice cream." The aim is to up the caloric density (the version above is about 300 calories) and find a recipe that a child is happy using daily. Shoot for 30 calories per ounce, which is about a third more calories per ounce than breast milk or formula. The same base can be used as a breakfast smoothie in which you put your child's tyrosine, carnosine, carnitine, or other amino acids that you are using therapeutically. Morning smoothies are also a great opportunity to add wake-up nutrients or herbs like B vitamins, inositol, or rhodiola.

A Natural Option: Goat Milk Infant Formula. This was the option that worked for my own son, who faltered on breast milk (even while I strictly avoided fish, shellfish, dairy, soy, eggs, all nuts, and some fruits), semi-elemental formulas, and soy formula. The recipe below is my own, and makes 8 ounces of formula that provide about 170 calories, 5–6 grams protein, 9–10 grams fat, and 10–11 grams carbohydrate. In one formula serving each day, add a dose of infant vitamin drops, such as Twin Labs Infant Care Multi. This is important since goat milk lacks some B vitamins crucial for babies. Let your pediatrician know if you plan to use this recipe, and be sure to monitor your baby's iron status with your doctor. Nutricia also makes a commercial goat milk infant formula called Karicare, more commonly available outside the United States.

> 5 ounces whole-fat goat milk
>
> 3 ounces water
>
> ¾ teaspoon flax oil (organic)
>
> ½ teaspoon safflower or sunflower oil (organic)
>
> 1½ teaspoons Lundberg brand organic brown rice syrup
>
> ⅛ teaspoon *Bifidobacterium infantis* probiotic powder, or a dusting of Klaire Labs Therbiotic Infant probiotic powder

Meyenberg powdered goat milk is convenient as it can be reconstituted as needed. Also, Karo syrup may be substituted for the brown rice syrup, if this is all that's available. Karo syrup is corn syrup.

A Controversial but Potentially Useful Test

Urine screening for polypeptides: This test is used to screen for inadequate digestion—*not* for allergy or inflammation—of wheat and dairy proteins in the diet. When these proteins are poorly digested, they may spill over into urine (according to a number of published studies) as long peptide fragments with neurotransmitter activity. These peptides also cross the blood-brain barrier, where they engage the same receptors that bind endorphins and opiate compounds—and where, some contend, they block expressive language, impair cognition, drive food cravings, trigger behavior swings, and lessen pain sensitivity. The original basis for gluten-free, casein-free diets for autism rests on the theory that removing these food proteins is the equivalent of withdrawing a brain-damaging opiate from the diet. Children have shown dramatic improvement with this measure, according to many anecdotal reports. Well-designed research remains to be done in the United States with this diet. So far, studies have been too weak and too poorly controlled in their design to clearly assess the effects of this diet. More information on this lab test and how to use gluten-free, casein-free diets can be found in *Special-Needs Kids Eat Right*.

This test remains controversial and is currently not covered by insurance. It costs about $100 and is available from Great Plains Laboratory (GreatPlainsLaboratory.com) and Genova Diagnostics (GenovaDiagnostics.com). It requires a urine sample. It may indicate whether or not your child would respond to a gluten-free, casein-free diet. Your child must be eating wheat, dairy, and soy foods regularly to get clear results (soy protein mimics milk protein on this test). Providers practicing biomedical interventions for autism will be familiar with this test, but others outside of that specialty may not.

Replenishment 101—For Parents

Chapter 2 of this book talks about helping your babies and kids sleep, but what about you? Moms and dads need sleep, too; to do that, you need to get your nutrients, rest, and TLC. Getting your baby to sleep is one thing. But don't overlook the fact that your own quality of sleep will be negatively impacted if you aren't taking care of *yourself*. It's not unusual for mothers to "lose" their normal sleep cycle after needing to get up frequently at night to care for a high-needs baby. Once baby is more settled, what about you? Don't neglect your own body chemistry to restore your ability to sleep—which is just as crucial for your health as it is for children. For kids and adults alike, several nutrients must work together to create the hormones, neurotransmitters, and overall comfortable constitution needed to sleep well. If your body just manufactured another human being, you need replenishment. If you are breast-feeding, definitely don't skimp on your own nutrients, especially healthful fats and oils, minerals, and protein. If you are the parent of a school-age or teenage special-needs child, you've had a more exhausting and depleting journey than parents of typical kids. You need to rebuild and restore, too. Use nutrition to boost your rest, brain, mood, health, and immunity. Here are a few top-of-the-list tips every pooped-out parent should consider:

• Take supplemental omega-3 fats. If your mood is low or you have mood swings, focus on EPA (an omega-3 fatty acid called eicosapentanoic acid) at 1–1.5 grams per day (that's grams, not milligrams). Use higher amounts of EPA relative to DHA (see the next paragraph). Lower doses are not likely to impact mood, but can be fine for overall good health (especially cardiac health); higher doses may be needed if you have intractable depression and mood swings. In that case, work with a mental health professional—don't neglect your own well-being. EPA has shown efficacy for bipolar disorder, and even for suicidality, at very high doses of 6 grams per day. A traditional Greenland Eskimo diet incorporates up to 14 grams of EPA with no toxic effects. These oils thin blood, so don't combine them with drugs such as Coumadin, warfarin, or daily high doses of aspirin without checking with your doctor. If you are planning a surgical procedure, stop taking blood-thinning fish oils a week before, or per your surgeon's instructions. They are compatible with most psychiatric medications, but always check with your doctor if you are adding a nutrient at doses that can have pharmacological effects. If EPA helps your mood and mood swings, know that abruptly stopping it may retrigger your symptoms, just as can be true with a medication.

• If you find you are having trouble with focus, attention, concentration, and memory, or if you are pregnant or nursing, the omega-3 oil to emphasize is DHA (docosahexasanoic acid). Take at least twice as much DHA relative to EPA. Besides fish oil supplements that provide more DHA than EPA (like DHA capsules from Nordic Naturals), sources for DHA include ground flaxseed, flax oil, walnuts or their oil, or hemp seed oil. These contain high amounts of alpha-linolenic acid, which is yet another fatty acid that we can *convert* to helpful DHA. But evidence has grown that we often don't do a very good job of this, and that infants may not do it adequately at all, which is why DHA is now added to formulas for babies. Using plant sources for DHA can work if you use a good-potency multivitamin (to make sure all nutrients needed to convert to DHA are aboard) and if you favor that conversion even more by eating more omega-3 oils (canola, flax, walnut) than omega-6 oils (safflower, sunflower, corn, soy, evening primrose, wheat germ). When using DHA as a supplement, start with at least 400 milligrams per day. When relying on vegetable sources, you will probably need about a tablespoon or two per day of flax oil, or about 4 grams daily of alpha-linolenic acid from all sources. If using ground flaxseed, know that high doses (more than 3 tablespoons per day) can interfere with thyroid function. The seed husks contain compounds that may inhibit uptake of iodine into the thyroid gland. Your doctor or naturopath can monitor thyroid function for you, if there is any question.

• There are dozens of fish oil supplement products. Read labels to make sure you are emphasizing the right omega-3 fatty acid for your needs (EPA for mood, DHA for focus and attention). Some have very little EPA and much more DHA in them, and vice versa. Most do not have enough oil in a single pill to be effective, so check the dose. Others simply say "1000 milligrams of omega-3 oils" or even "1000 milligrams of fish oil" without telling exactly which oils are in there, or how much. This is no bargain—you need to know how much EPA and DHA you are getting. For mood benefits, you need more than twice as much EPA in your supplement as DHA. A good product for this is Coromega, or EPA capsules from Nordic Naturals. Visit Omega-Direct.com for an easy glance at the array of products available from Nordic Naturals. If you scroll over a product image, it will flash EPA and DHA content for you. Visit the Coromega website for a unique gel formulation that many kids like, with flavors such as chocolate orange and lime. Another reputable maker of fish oil is Pharmax, which is usually sold through health care providers.

• Two great books on these oils are *The Omega-3 Connection* by Andrew Stoll, MD (2001), and *The LCP Solution* by Jacqueline Stordy, PhD (2001).

- Use a good calcium plus magnesium supplement. It should:

  ▪ Provide 400–800 milligrams per day of magnesium, possibly more depending on your diet. If it triggers loose stools, back down on the magnesium level, take a lower dose at two or three intervals rather than lots all at once, or use a less laxative form (magnesium citrate is more laxative while magnesium glycinate is usually less so).

  ▪ Provide calcium from mixed sources, not just calcium carbonate. Calcium carbonate buffers stomach acid. You need acid in your stomach to initiate normal digestion. Over time, buffering your stomach on a daily basis may diminish digestion, enzyme output, and absorption of all nutrients. It can also create an imbalance in calcium chemistry, such that calcium is pulled from bone and redeposited in the wrong places as oxalate stones, such as kidney tissue or joints.

  ▪ Your total calcium intake daily should be around 1200 milligrams, unless your doctor has instructed you otherwise.

  ▪ If you must use calcium carbonate, use it with meals and food, not on an empty stomach. Reflux medications may impair calcium absorption (and that of other minerals as well).

  ▪ Calcium and magnesium can help sleep. Adults and children can use this supplement near bedtime, to further support good sleep.

- Use a high-potency multivitamin that gives you a full complement of all B-group vitamins, and at least half your daily value for minerals such as iron, zinc, selenium, and chromium. All these vitamins and minerals are needed to run the metabolic machinery that makes proteins, hormones, tissues, and neurotransmitters; releases toxins; and much more.

• It's stating the obvious to tell you to feed yourself well, but you should. Slow-cooked stews and roasts are easy to make and can be filled with protein, fiber, and mineral-rich organic meats, vegetables, and fresh herbs. Get a slow cooker or pressure cooker, or try time-bake with convection on your oven to cook fresh whole foods faster, while retaining their nutrients more. Slow cookers and oven roasters let you combine everything in your recipe in the morning and simmer it slowly all day. This is an easy family dinner strategy that can usually accommodate special diet needs. Set up meals that use fresh whole ingredients on your schedule. Potatoes, beets, carrots, yams, sweet potatoes, green or wax beans, and winter squashes cook quickly in pressure cookers, and the taste is worth it over frozen or canned versions of these foods. Slow-baked or roasted chicken, beef, or pork is delicious and easy to prepare, too.

• If you are back to menstruating again after birth, or having periods that last more than four days soaking more than a pad an hour, you may be anemic. Anemia makes you cranky, tired, easily winded, and forgetful. It impairs your immune response, triggers poor sleep, and lowers appetite. The more anemic you are, the heavier your monthly bleeding can be. Heavier, more frequent periods are common as we approach menopause, and this is depleting, as is providing full nourishment to your baby every day from your own body through breast milk. Have your doctor check your hemoglobin, hematocrit, and ferritin levels. If you need an iron supplement, try easy-to-absorb forms such as ferrous bis-glycinate or food source tablets such as MegaFood Blood Builder rather than the usual ferrous sulfate tablets that doctors prescribe. If you need large doses daily (doctors may prescribe 80–100 milligrams per day for certain circumstances), you can use these products in split doses to improve tolerance and prevent constipation sometimes triggered by taking large doses of iron. Take with food, especially vitamin C–containing foods or acidic foods such as tomato sauce or orange juice. If you eat meat, treat yourself to some organic grass-fed beef from a local source to minimize contamination from bacteria or agricultural chemicals. The iron in red muscle tissue is the most bioavailable of all and will help you rebuild your blood.

• Haven't heard the news yet on vitamin D? Then you probably *are* under a rock, and need some sunshine! In 2005, a review released in the *Journal of Nutrition* stated that most people in North America are vitamin D depleted or deficient. Most vulnerable among us are persons living in the more northerly states, the elderly especially, and persons with darker pigmented skin. Vitamin D is a nutrient critical for much more than we previously appreciated. It has hormone-like behavior in the body, and plays a role in multiple disease states, mood and depression, respiratory infection and flu prevention, and bone health. It may be a better preventive for flu than flu vaccine, according to emerging research. Low vitamin D status correlates with higher risk for several cancers. We can convert sunlight to vitamin D through a chemical reaction in the skin, but people with dark skin need more time in sunlight to create enough vitamin D. Depending on the weather and where you live, just a few minutes of sunshine (without sunscreen) daily can help vitamin D status, but it is now recommended that you also take vitamin D supplements. Adults need at least 2000 and possibly 5000 international units per day, and this is easily had in small gel caps or concentrated vitamin D3 drops. Most doctors are on board with this news and will know to supplement you if your vitamin D level is below 40 nanomoles/L or 16 nanograms/L. If you are really depleted, you may need a weekly dose of tens of thousands of international units (IUs) of vitamin D and your doctor can help you with this. Vitamin D toxicity is low. Small children can take 1000 international units per day, and older kids and teens may need up to 5000 international units per day. This is especially important when they live in darker, cooler climates and rarely get outside.

• If postpartum depression is plaguing you, or you are depleted from years of battle with school districts, child care providers, contentious relatives, special medical needs, budget challenges, and so on, use all the tools at your disposal to cope and feel better. Nutrition-focused tools can be part of your support system. These can include the same ones a child may use for mood, depression, anxiety, and depletion, tailored to your adult weight and individual context for health concerns. Common supplements for mood include serotonin boosters such as 5-hydroxytryptophan, tyrosine, Saint John's wort, and many other nutrients. For specific instructions on safely using these and other nutrition supports for yourself, see *The Mood Cure* by Julia Ross. Just as you would for your child, if you'd like to use some of these tools, talk with an experienced health professional about dosing, and don't mix with prescription drugs without guidance.

• Last but certainly not least, buy the most pristine and nutritious food you can afford, as often as possible. I am an unabashed proponent of locally sourced, organic foods, including meats, chicken, eggs, cheese, milk, and produce. Three reasons: (1) Some organic food crops show better nutrient profiles than conventionally raised crops, for protein quality, vitamins, and minerals. (2) The closer you are to the source, the fresher and more nutritious your food will be. (3) Americans eat about 3 pounds of pesticides annually, not to mention about 28 micrograms of mercury daily (about the amount in a flu shot), plus unknown amounts of endocrine-triggering residues from plastic packaging. Americans also eat a lot more genetically modified foods and colorings, flavorings, and additives than residents of most other developed countries, where many of these items are banned owing to a lack of research on their long-term effects. Why opt to eat known carcinogens if you don't have to? Many agricultural pesticides are lipophilic, meaning they like to be surrounded by fat molecules. These may concentrate in the fat of your milk if you are breast-feeding, *your* liver, kidney, and brain tissue if you aren't, and your baby's brain, liver, and kidneys, too. Fats are essential to your baby's brain growth, nerve cell function, and development. Your special-needs baby does not need another battle to fight, so don't feed her pesticides or chemicals that may interfere with gene expression, hormone signaling, or the capacity to excrete toxins in her delicate metabolism.

Remembering that our children deserve wellness, even when they have special needs, is important. While there is literally more bad news than ever before about the state of health for U.S. children today, you can change the course of this for your own child by integrating sound nutrition strategies. Seek out the tools and providers who help you on this path, and you may be surprised and pleased by the results.

Index

About the Author

Judy Converse, MPH, RD, LD, is a licensed registered dietician with graduate and undergraduate degrees in nutrition. Since 1999, she has worked in private practice with children of all ages who have developmental delay, autism, allergy, asthma, or intractable issues with behavior, learning, feeding, growth, or mood. After working in outpatient health maintenance and sustainable/organic foods awareness, Ms. Converse's career path took a change of course when she became a parent and saw that there was little to be had at the pediatrician's office for concrete nutrition support and advice. She has since worked with families, government agencies, and special-needs nonprofit organizations to inform on how to use evidence-based nutrition strategies for a gamut of pediatric health and wellness concerns, from how to help babies and toddlers sleep and eat better to how to effectively use special diets for autism. Ms. Converse has written several articles on nutrition care for children with autism and has lectured to both professional and parent audiences on this topic. In 2008, she published the first professionally accredited learning module on nutrition and special diet strategies for autism, "Medical Nutrition Therapy for Pediatric Autism: Strategies for Assessment and Monitoring," to help providers in the pediatric autism community understand the powerful role of nutrition and diets in this developmental dilemma. A New England native, Ms. Converse currently lives in Colorado with her husband and son.